Secrets to Surgery Success:

TAKE CHARGE & HEAL FASTER

A Comprehensive Step-by-Step Guide
to Achieving Peak Health for Surgery

By Susan S. Wilder, MD, IFMCP,
CEO LifeScape Premier & LifeScape Health Ventures

www.optimizesurgery.com and www.lifescapepremier.com

Copyright 2020
LifeScape Health Ventures

ISBN 13: 979-8-5984310-1-6

Book Description

Just as anyone would be foolish to run a marathon without training, you would be equally unwise to face surgery without preparing. *Surgery is the most significant athletic event most of us will ever face.* In **Secrets to Surgery Success,** and the online program **optimizesurgery.com,** Dr. Wilder distills decades of medical and functional medicine experience along with extensive research guiding you through simple modules to optimize your physical, mental and emotional health and provides strategies to adopt habits that support a smooth surgery and rapid recovery.

Surgery is risky. However, every patient chooses whether to engage proactively or passively, as a warrior or victim. Surgical complications are common, costly, sometimes fatal, yet often avoidable. Complications occur in over one third of surgeries, far more than previously estimated. Upwards of 40% of surgical deaths are preventable. Complications cost in myriad ways including prolonged hospitalization, mounting medical bills that may run from thousands to over a million dollars, delayed return to work and life, permanent disability or disfigurement, and death.

Most approach surgery passively, assuming the surgeon and his or her team will handle everything necessary to assure the best outcome. Physicians know that required "preoperative clearances" have never proven to improve outcomes. Excellent care taken by surgical teams fails to address ***the most important contributor to surgical outcomes…the patient's state of health*** on entering the operating room.

Clinically proven strategies offer patients significant control over surgical outcomes. Armed with inspiration and strategies to transform your health, you can increase your chances of a successful surgery and uneventful recovery. Those who stick with the strategies taught in this program are likely to find their health transformed for life.

This book and online program are dedicated to Leo, whose love and wisdom we greatly miss, and to all who have suffered needlessly. May their lessons inspire and empower us to prevent similar fates for others.

Great losses are great lessons

Contents

Book Description iii
Introduction: Why I Created This Program 1
What Makes This Program Unique 7
What to Expect In Secrets To Surgery Success? 9
Who Will Benefit From This Program? 13
A Special Message For Surgeons 16

Chapter 1: Optimizing Healing:
    Lifestyle and Nutrition Strategy 23
Chapter 2: Optimizing Detoxification:
    Prepping The Liver And GI Tract For Surgery 36
Chapter 3: Mentally Preparing For Surgery 49
Chapter 4: Reducing Complications After Surgery 64
Chapter 5: Musculoskeletal Fitness For Surgery:
    Assuring Healthy Muscles, Bones, Tendons And Joints . . 70
Chapter 6: Optimizing Recovery:
    Clear Toxins, Control Pain, Boost Healing & Promote
    Immune Function 79
Chapter 7: Vitality Beyond Surgery 93

Appendix 1: Am I A Good Surgical Candidate? 97
Appendix 2: Starting Point Metrics 99
Appendix 3: Daily Habit Checklist 101
Appendix 4: Hidden Dangers In Your Medicine Cabinet 103
Appendix 5: Common Surgical Complications, Preventive
    Strategies, & When To Seek Help 107
Appendix 6: Mindset for Intention 124
Appendix 7: Meditation Before Surgery 126
Appendix 8: Resources For Additional Support 129
    Other Resources (U.S.) 132
Appendix 9: Simple Healing Recipes 134

References 138
Acknowledgements 142
About The Author 144

Introduction:
Why I Created This Program

As a Family Physician Certified in Functional Medicine, I am passionate about PREVENTION. Sadly, Americans now boast the worst collective health metrics and longevity of any economically advanced nation, including a several year *decline* in life expectancy! Children born in the United States today are likely to experience more years of chronic disease and disability and die younger than those in other economically advanced nations. True to our priorities, our medical system achieves the poorest overall health results in the developed world at the highest cost, mainly because we emphasize rescue over prevention. Think about it. We spend whatever it takes to treat a cancer, open blocked arteries, throw a slew of expensive drugs at every symptom, scramble to manage a predicted pandemic or institutionalize an Alzheimer's victim, yet we spend less than 3% of our health care dollar preventing those very problems, and they are very preventable.

We each take our health for granted…until it fails. Functional medicine revived my health, resolving years of chronic fatigue, fibromyalgia, hormone issues and infertility, depression, chronic neck pain, acid reflux, and arthritis simply by addressing their root causes and taking action. Undergoing surgery when I was a hot mess was disastrous. I suffered significant brain fog and chronic memory issues after surgery because I did not realize, even as a physician, that my genetics, diet, medications, toxic exposures, sleep habits and poor stress management significantly impaired my ability to recover from the effects of drugs like anesthetics and pain medications.

I vow to keep YOU or your loved ones from suffering that same fate, or worse. When we delve into root causes of chronic symptoms and take action to resolve them, diseases we understood to be irreversible suddenly IMPROVE or even RESOLVE.

Chronic disease need NOT be a life sentence!

Root causes we will explore include dietary and nutritional deficiencies, toxin exposures through food, water, air or medicines, food or environmental allergies or intolerances, stress, sleep problems, lack of activity, and genetics. In genomics we say that genes load the weapon, but environment (our choices and our habits) pulls the trigger. Remember, just because something runs in your family does not mean you are doomed to the same fate. We don't just hand down genes, we also hand down habits.

Today, I am literally decades younger and healthier than I was when I left a prestigious position at one of the nation's premier academic medical institutions to found LifeScape in 2003. Since then, I have witnessed hundreds of similar brilliant health breakthroughs and I know this is also possible for YOU.

Surgery is a risky undertaking, too often taken without much thought or preparation. We might run a few tests to see if you are safe to undergo surgery – none of which are proven to reduce risk of complications or improve likelihood of recovery. However, you have more control than you think over your state of health, mind, body, and spirit heading into surgery as well as how smooth and quick your recovery will be.

During surgery, you receive anesthesia, which suppresses your consciousness and breathing ability. Anesthesiologists and nurse anesthetists do a brilliant job taking control of your brain and bodily functions while keeping you sedated. Your health, or lack thereof, determines how effectively you process those drugs. After surgery, you may need pain medications and other medicines that can cause side effects and complications. Too many of us have livers clogged with fat or inundated by chronic toxins including alcohol, acetaminophen, narcotics, hormones, environmental toxins, or other medicines. We may also have colons clogged by fiber-poor diets. Too many suffer from nutrient deficiencies and poor immune and gut function from decades of eating a standard American diet (with the apt acronym, S.A.D.) full of refined, highly processed foods and sugars, without enough fiber or critical plant-based phytonutrients (found in greens and colorful vegetables). Acid blockers, antibiotics, hormones, herbicides/pesticides in food, and pain medications devastate our gut microbiome – millions of microbes that serve as command and control center for clearing toxins and managing immune, hormone, and brain function. In any ecosystem, including that of the human body, diversity is key to resilience. Unfortunately, microbial diversity in the average American is now, on average, a pathetic fraction of what is considered optimal.

Decades of physical inactivity leave many of us with weak muscles, unstable or stiff joints, poor balance, and poor circulation. Excessive stress, poor sleep and insufficient hydration round out the common reasons most of us are chronically sick and tired. If this sounds like you, this program will not only help you cruise through surgery and heal quickly, it has the potential to help you achieve your own life-changing brilliant health breakthrough.

This book and the online program (at optimizesurgery.com) compiles decades of research and experience managing the most common surgical mishaps and considering preventive measures that might have helped. It includes insights from surgeons, anesthesiologists, oncologists, and physical therapists. I have sadly lost patients and loved ones to preventable deaths, and those losses fuel my passion for helping you achieve your best outcome possible. Studies show that more than 40% of surgical deaths and an even higher percentage of complications are preventable. In health, you always have a choice:

Do you intend to be a passive victim or an active warrior?

Secrets to Surgery Success is a comprehensive, evidence-based, easy to navigate guide to help you understand surgical risks and avert them as much as humanly possible while gradually shifting your health for the better. This program cannot guarantee a good outcome nor does any of this replace or override the guidance of your medical team. My goal is simply to give you the tools and the knowledge with which to actively take control of your health and enhance your medical team's efforts.

I guarantee treasuring your health does not need to be difficult, boring, or full of sacrifice. *Small steps practiced consistently over time create massive impact.* Pay attention to the side effects of feeling energized and looking amazing. Sadly, most of us have no idea what truly good health feels like – many have never experienced it. What do you have to lose? You can see results in even a few weeks of concerted effort.

Honor yourself and treasure your health by engaging in Secrets to Surgery Success or, for a more in-depth audiovisual course, its online program Preparing for Surgery at optimizesurgery.com.

Working hard for something we don't care about is called stress... working hard for something we love is called passion

Simon Sinek

What Makes This Program Unique

Secrets to Surgery Success is truly revolutionary in applying decades of clinical knowledge, research, and experience from allopathic medicine with evidence-proven strategies from functional and integrative medicine.

If you engage actively and consistently, you can expect to gain:

- Appreciation of your health & a commitment to be a better steward of it
- Reduced reliance on medications by understanding healthy non-drug responses to common symptoms
- Understanding of surgical and postoperative risks and specific strategies to avert them
- Understanding of what to monitor for after surgery
- Understanding of the impact of lifestyle choices around diet, hydration, movement, stress management, attitude, and sleep on overall health
- A positive mindset around surgery and health in general
- Improved GI tract function

- Improved overall mood, energy, vitality
- Mindful recognition of specific habits or choices that created health problems

What to Expect In Secrets To Surgery Success?

Where Do I Begin?

Congratulations on taking the first step to treasuring your health.

Although this book focuses on preparing you to cruise through surgery and recover quickly and fully, I truly hope you will take the strategies learned here beyond surgery.

Pay attention to how your body feels when you treat it with the reverence it deserves and commit to moving forward with habits that pay off for you. Note which habits that make you feel more energized and vibrant or help you achieve better sleep and mood. What happens when you revert to old habits? Learning to tune in and listen to your body is life changing.

So where do we begin?

FIRST note your surgery date and set a Preparing for Surgery start date at least 2-4 weeks prior. The more lead-time, the better your ability to achieve the best health possible.

NEXT, complete the "Am I a Good Surgical Candidate" survey (see Appendix 1) and score it. If you score 0-2, congratulations, you are ahead of the curve so keep up the good work. If, like most of us, you score 3 or greater, then pay close attention to all the strategies offered throughout this program. Consider investing in recommended supplements to support your digestive tract and healthy gut bacteria to get your system in high gear to handle the toxic insults of surgery. If you score 10 or more, I strongly encourage you to schedule a virtual or in-person appointment with one of our nutritionist/health coaches or book a comprehensive functional medicine consultation with one of our expert providers to delve deeply into resuscitating an extremely stressed or neglected system (www.lifescapepremier.com).

THIRD, copy your Starting Point and Daily Habit Checklist into a daily journal or print for use leading to surgery (see Appendix 2) enter your starting metrics, your health commitment and your WHY. For health commitment to stick, you must define WHY this focus on your health is so critical.

FOURTH, order your supplements to support detoxification and healing and start taking them at least 2 weeks prior to surgery (https://bit.ly/2RbQqel).

FINALLY get rolling with Chapter 1 and progress through the program at a pace that will keep you on track for surgery.

Most important, invest at least 5 minutes each day to focus entirely on you. Use the morning ritual, daily meditation, and habit checklist to keep you moving forward mindfully and gratefully.

Be gentle with yourself, understanding that perfection is NOT the goal. Building habits takes time, patience, and practice. Recognize when you fall back into habits that are not serving you. As they say, first step in getting out a hole is to quit digging.

Notice mindfully and without judgement when cravings sabotage you. Try to create an environment at home and work that facilitates healthier choices. Notify your friends, family, and coworkers about what you are doing and why and engage their support. Give yourself permission to be imperfect, consider what triggered the slip, and gently recommit to getting back on track and working towards the goal of finding your best health.

Enjoy the journey!

You yourself, as much as anybody in the entire universe, deserve your love and affection

Buddha

Who Will Benefit From This Program?

Preparing for Surgery is perfect for you if:

- you, or someone you care about, are anticipating surgery in the next year, or even in the next month
- you like to be prepared, know what to expect, and how to maximize your odds of success
- you know someone who has suffered surgical complications and want to avoid them for yourself
- you lost someone you knew and are extremely anxious or fearful about surgery
- you want a safe surgery and to exceed even your surgeon's expectations for recovery
- you cannot afford "down time" and must heal quickly to get back in action
- you are sick and tired of feeling unhealthy – lethargic, overweight, or suffering from chronic pain, or chronic disabling diseases such as arthritis, heart or lung disease, diabetes or cancer
- you want to look and feel better – active, glowing, vibrant

- you realize that surgery treats a symptom, but your overall, long-term health relies on your choices
- you treasure your health and are willing to invest in optimizing it
- you are ready to change things up and start revising habits that are failing you
- you want to prepare mentally and physically to assure you are in your best mindset for surgery
- you want to prevent future surgeries by addressing root causes
- you want to commit to being an active warrior for your health, rather than a passive victim
- your goal is not simply to survive, but THRIVE

I will prevent disease whenever I can, for prevention is preferable to cure

Hippocrates

A Special Message For Surgeons

As I stated in my last speech to graduating residents and fellows as a Mayo Residency Director in 2002, "if a prescription pad or a scalpel are the only tools in your arsenal, you will win a few battles, but you will lose the war."

I have devoted over half my career to studying and practicing functional or root cause medicine. When we address the biochemical, social, mental and emotional root causes of chronic symptoms, diseases we consider irreversible magically RESOLVE including arthritis, type 2 diabetes (which consumes an inordinate percentage of our healthcare dollar), high blood pressure, asthma, autoimmune diseases like lupus, and neurologic disorders like headaches, attention deficit, mood disorders and memory problems. Root causes we explore include nutrient deficiencies, toxin exposures through food, drugs, water, or air; food or environmental allergies or intolerances, stress, sleep problems, lack of activity, and, of course, genetics.

As a surgeon, your dedication to the art and practice of surgery is truly admirable and I know your work is progressively more complex and challenging. In just a generation, our patient population has become progressively sicker with more chronic health issues, more immune dysfunction, escalating obesity and increasing dependency on chronic medications. American citizens are over-medicated and under-well. The very term *"chronic disease management"* is a travesty. As one of my patients noted, *"my other doctors just monitor my deterioration."* Even our lab "norms" have morphed to that of an unhealthy population. Ideal fasting glucose is 65-80, yet the lab parameters do not flag abnormal until over 100, a point at which immune function and surgical healing are potentially impaired. With the majority of our population now overweight or obese and over 130 million diabetic or pre-diabetic, it is rare to see a truly "ideal" fasting blood sugar anymore.

You prepare intensively for every case and I designed this program to support your efforts, coaching your patients through steps to optimize every facet of their health in advance of surgery. The goal is to get motivated patients literally training for surgery, ostensibly the greatest athletic event of their lives. Preoperative clearances, to assess safety to undergo surgery, have never proven to reduce risk of complications nor improve likelihood of excellent outcomes.

Imagine how great it would be if your patients entered the operating room in their best condition possible, immune system optimized, liver and gut primed to detoxify, lungs strengthened, clot risks mitigated, and mentally and emotionally geared to enter surgery with a positive mindset, reducing their need for risky anxiolytics and narcotic pain medicines.

I personally suffered significant brain fog and irreversible memory issues after a fairly minor skin cancer surgery because

17

I did not realize, even as a physician, how my genetics, chronic medications, nutrient-poor diet, insufficient sleep or stress management strategies significantly impaired my ability to clear toxins. Too many suffer from nutrient deficiencies, inflammation, poor immune and gut function from decades of eating a standard American diet (or S.A.D.) full of refined and processed foods and sugars, woefully inadequate in fiber or plant-based phytonutrients. Chronic acid blockers, antibiotics and other medications wreak havoc on our gut microbiome – the command and control center for detoxification and immune, hormone, and neurotransmitter function. Acid blockers, among the most commonly prescribed medications, also impair nutrient absorption and increase risk of pneumonia and c. difficile colitis, complications we all hope to avoid. Too many of us suffer weak muscles and stiff or unstable joints from decades of inactivity and nutrient-poor diets. Excessive stress, poor sleep and insufficient water intake round out the common reasons most of us are chronically sick and tired. This program will not only help your patients cruise through surgery and heal spectacularly, it has the potential to help any participant achieve their own life-changing brilliant health breakthrough.

I've spent decades researching and witnessing the most common surgical mishaps, interviewing surgeons and anesthesiologists, nutritionists and physical therapists, and rehashing adverse outcomes and examining what we could have done differently. I have sadly lost patients and loved ones whose deaths were likely preventable, and those losses fuel my passion for helping you help your patients. Studies show that more than 40% of surgical deaths and the vast majority of complications are preventable.

Preparing for Surgery is a comprehensive, evidence-based guide to educate your patients and provide them with tools and simple strategies to maximize health. Modules covered include:

- Diet and Lifestyle
- Optimizing Detoxification
- Mentally Preparing for Surgery
- Strategies to Reduce Surgical Complications
- Fitness for Surgery
- Optimizing Recovery

Preparing for Surgery also suggests a few supplements that do not increase bleeding or blood clot risk and have no significant risk of drug interaction. The program reviews all medications and supplements that are critical to avoid peri-operatively given bleeding, drug interaction or surgical risk. The evidence-based supplement protocol simply supports biochemical processes for hepatic and gastrointestinal detoxification, wound healing and resolution of bruising, gastric motility, and immune optimization. We clearly reiterate, this program cannot guarantee a good outcome nor does any of this replace or override your guidance or that of their medical team. Preparing for Surgery supports your efforts by offering your patients the tools and knowledge to take their health to another level.

As our modern Hippocratic Oath states:

"I will apply, for the benefit of the sick, all measures [that] are required, avoiding those twin traps of overtreatment and therapeutic nihilism.

I will remember that there is art to medicine as well as science, and that warmth, sympathy, and understanding may outweigh the surgeon's knife or the chemist's drug...

I will prevent disease whenever I can, for prevention is preferable to cure."

A Special Message For Surgeons

Every new day is a chance to change your life

Chapter 1:

Optimizing Healing: Lifestyle And Nutrition Strategy

Illustrative Story

The Reluctant Warrior – Never Too Late to Take Ownership of Your Health

I felt it, along with a sinking feeling in my gut—the firm, fixed mass, hard as a rock, in the neck of a patient I was examining for the very first time. My fears came to life as a biopsy confirmed the mass to be lymphoma requiring urgent surgical resection. George was in his late 70s, the culmination of a lifetime of neglected health resulting in a litany of chronic conditions that put him at very high risk for surgical complications. Fortunately, his wife, who chided, "lack of self care is SO selfish," successfully nagged him into getting a physical and thereby saved his life. No wonder married men live longer!

George's issues included obesity, uncontrolled diabetes with fasting blood sugars over 180, inflammation with a C-reactive protein measurement over 10, high blood pressure in the 160-170s/90-100s and elevated liver enzymes indicating a liver likely clogged with fat. His diet was the typical S.A.D. (short for the Standard American Diet), including carb-loaded breakfast *of juice, toast or bagels, and cereal, lunches and dinners were heavy on sandwiches, burgers and fries, meat and potatoes, or processed foods including processed luncheon meats (known to be cancer-promoting). He drank mostly coffee, beer with golf, nightly cocktails, and enjoyed frequent desserts. Fruits, vegetables and fiber were woefully deficient from his daily habit. Like many Americans, he was consuming at least 20 tsp of added sugars per day, more than twice the recommended limit. (Men: 150 calories **per day** (37.5 grams or 9 teaspoons) Women: 100 calories **per day** (25 grams or 6 teaspoons).*

Obesity alone put him at very high risk. No surgeon wants to operate on an obese patient because of the technical difficulty entailed, plus a 5-fold increased risk of heart attacks, 4-fold increased risk of nerve injury and higher risk of blood clots, lung complications and infections. Adding insult to injury, diabetes put George at particular risk because high blood sugar effectively paralyzes immune function, rendering our defense against cancer and infection helpless. He quickly needed his blood sugar normalized to heal from surgery and his immune system fully engaged to fight his cancer.

George was not particularly motivated to change his lifestyle, and rebelled after being nudged to undergo a physical that put him on a roller coaster careening toward his own mortality. His mindset was fixated in passive victim mode; "Just cut this tumor out and give me some pills," he said, "and I'll be fine." However, he was into cars, so I used the high performance vehicle analogy to help him understand that he was fueling his high performance vehicle with garbage, damaging the fuel injector (insulin) and leaving toxic waste clogging the engine. However, if he adopted a few simple changes, we could quickly help him get back into the race, and stave off disability and death by taking aggressive action immediately.

I started him on medication for diabetes and high blood pressure (reminding him we could taper these as his diet and health improved), and supplements to support blood sugar control, immune function, and clear his clogged liver. He added 4oz of an organic greens juice blend twice daily, changed breakfast to appetite-satisfying protein + healthy fat. He learned about healthy portions, eliminated sodas easily, limited dessert to weekends and committed to 1 large salad or veggie-full soup, chili, or stir fry daily to further boost his vegetable intake. He cut alcohol (another carcinogen) to half his previous intake—removing it altogether in the weeks leading up to surgery—breaking his nightly habit. Within 2 weeks his fasting blood sugar was under 100, his CRP inflammatory marker was <2, his weight was down 8lb, his liver enzymes improved, and his blood pressure was controlled. His wife commented on his remarkably improved energy level and mood, saying, "He's a new man!" He enjoyed better sleep, a revived sex drive, and noted he no longer needed acid blockers for frequent acid reflux. Eliminating reflux and acid-blockers dramatically reduced his pneumonia risk.

In his 70's, George had transformed from being a passive victim to an active warrior for his health. His surgery successfully cured his lymphoma and, 10 years later, George remained cancer-free with a healthy liver, heart and brain because he retained several of the simple health habits that supported him through surgery.

Health is our most important asset, yet we often neglect or fail to appreciate it until it falters. Opting for instant gratification over long-term stewardship and for rescue over prevention leads to failure – and our nation boasts the dismal health and health cost statistics to show for it.

The core of this program is *Stewardship, defined as*:

The careful and responsible management of something entrusted to one's care.

We are responsible for our health – not our parents, family, schools, doctors, employers, health plans or government.

Just imagine what our world would be like if every one of us took personal responsibility to heart?

By engaging in this program, you are not only committing to preparing yourself for surgery, you are creating the potential to improve the trajectory of your health... should you choose to accept the challenge.

Life is all about choices.

Our choices about what we eat and drink, how we sleep, move, manage stress, and even what we think determine whether we experience decades of chronic disease, early disability and shortened life or whether we experience a vibrant health span.

As we begin the process of optimizing health for surgery, it is important to think about the root causes of chronic disease. If we dig up the roots, disease withers. If we simply medicate the symptoms and fail to address the root causes, disease will keep erupting in different ways.

Let me give you an example. Arguably, poor nutrition is the most common root cause of chronic disease. Consider that a standard American diet, full of processed, chemically-laden, food-like products, excessive sugar, refined starches, animal proteins, and unhealthy fats and woefully insufficient in critical plant-based nutrients, fiber, and healthy fats. In addition, mineral depletion of our soils over the past 100 years has resulted in even our healthy fruits, vegetables, and dairy products possessing drastically diminished amounts of their previous nutrient content. Commonly our day consists of a breakfast of juice, refined/processed herbicide-contaminated cereal, hormone-tainted milk, lunches of sandwiches, burgers, chips or fries, and excessive carbohydrate and protein-heavy dinners. Top it off with more processed or fructose-filled drinks, snacks and alcohol. On this diet, we first might notice weight gain and an unhealthy spare tire around our waist. This is never healthy, even in children. Then hormone issues and acne emerge for which a doctor might prescribe medicines. Next thing you know you feel lethargic or even depressed, leading to yet more medicine and costly tests. Then high blood pressure, blood sugar and arthritis emerge…leading to more and more drugs prescribed; and ultimately cancer, heart attacks, stroke. If you survive those, dementia or Parkinson's will emerge, rendering you disabled for your "golden years."

You get the picture of how one root cause can branch into multiple negative outcomes. Treating each symptom in the standard "pill-for-an-ill" medical approach might provide a temporary Band-aid, but you are ultimately playing whack-amole. If you fail to clean up your diet, you will find yourself on a slew of medications and progressively worse problems will inevitably surface.

YOU can control the root causes of the vast majority of our chronic diseases, including nutrient deficiencies, insufficient sleep, stress, a sedentary lifestyle, toxin exposures, and food allergies and sensitivities. This is great, because it means YOU ARE IN CONTROL. Remember, genes are not your destiny. Our genes just load the weapon...our choices pull the trigger.

Think about it. How many of our inherited ailments are in reality inherited habits? We could eliminate over 75% of preventable disease by following just FIVE Pillars of Healthy Lifestyle:

1. Sit less and get physically active at least 30 minutes most days (150minutes/week)
2. Avoid tobacco exposure of any kind
3. Maintain an ideal weight and waist circumference less than your hips (under 35"/89cm for a woman, 40"/101.6cm for a man)
4. Consume a diet rich in fruits and vegetables
5. Minimize red meat, sweetened beverages, refined and processed foods

Sadly, only 3% of the American population can claim all five!

Over three decades practicing medicine taught me that we are not logical beings. Most of us know what we SHOULD be doing, so how do we shift from SHOULD to MUST?

First, you MUST be CRYSTAL CLEAR on your WHY. Why is prioritizing your health important to you? After thinking through at least five levels of whys, you can achieve clarity and have a shot at your own brilliant health breakthrough!

Core Lifestyle and Nutrition Strategies to begin the process:

- COMMIT to treasuring your health every day – affirm with a daily mindset meditation, mantra, or prayer
- CREATE your environment for success – at home, work, school or sports - eliminate traps, avalanche foods (those foods you know you eat mindlessly and cannot stop), dump hidden junk food, and distractions that derail your journey to health
- COLLABORATE with those close to you and seek their...
- COMMITMENT to support your journey rather than sabotage your efforts
- CLEAN up your diet
- DITCH junk foods, fast food, sodas and juices
- HYDRATE. Drink at least 64oz or half your weight in filtered water daily. Infuse it with fruit, cucumber, mint, or mix it up with coffee, tea (green, white, herbal, hibiscus, dandelion), sparkling, mineral or tonic water with a little lemon or lime, or wholesome organic broths for variety
- Eat a whole foods diet rich in colorful fruits and vegetables

29

- Eat foods your great-grandmother would recognize
- Shop the periphery of the grocery store or check out farmer's markets or co-ops

As food author Michael Pollan stated,

"Eat real food, mostly plants, not too much" ...and "If it's delivered through your car window, it's not food"

- Aim for at least 3 cups greens, 3 cups colorful veggies daily and some legumes – beans, peas, lentils and whole grains for fiber if tolerated
- Eat the rainbow – a meal devoid of color, mostly white or brown, leaves your body STARVING for critical nutrients. Phyto- or plant-based nutrients are critical for building healthy tissues, hormones, brain chemicals and virtually every function of your body
- Try to eat organic for the Dirty Dozen most pesticide-laden foods: https://www.ewg.org/foodnews/dirty-dozen.php
- Try the 5S strategy to boost vegetable intake...aim for at least one veggie-laden Smoothie, Soup, Salad, Stew or chili, Stir-fry or bowl each meal
- Aim for 3 parts or handfuls of vegetables to every part of animal protein

- Use short cuts such as organic greens drinks or powders, frozen organic smoothie or fruit packets, or any of a number of pre-made organic plant-based fresh or frozen meals
- Stockpile a freezer full of easy microwavable healthy soups, chili, bowls and meals for after surgery
- Use small plates – you consume 30% fewer calories using salad plates instead of dinner plates – this simple habit can help you shed a pound a week
- Consider time-restricted eating (limiting any caloric foods or drinks to 8 hours daily) or intermittent fasting. In the past 40 years, Americans have added an average of 500 calories, or a full extra meal, to our daily intake fueling the twin epidemics of obesity and diabetes. Fasting at least 3 hours before bed, and 12 hours overnight is critical to preventing insulin resistance, a key root cause of diabetes, cardiovascular risk, osteoporosis and dementia. Extending that fast to 18 hours per day, even just 2-3 days per week, is a super simple way to improve metabolism and blood sugar. Exciting research reveals that regular fasting has powerful anti-aging and brain preserving impacts
- Include a little healthy fat with each meal, such as high-quality extra virgin olive oil, avocado, organic nut butters or nuts and seeds if tolerated, and wild caught fatty fish. Snack on organic nuts, seeds or trail mix. Organic ground flaxseed or chia seeds add healthy fat to smoothies, oatmeal, baked goods or purees. Healthy fats suppress your appetite helping you feel full longer, maintain the

health of every cell, keep your brain and nervous system sharp, help you absorb key nutrients, produce hormones and clear toxins
- Eat healthy lean proteins in small portions (nuts, seeds, legumes, wild-caught fish, organic poultry/ eggs/ dairy, grass-fed beef). A portion for animal protein is the size of a deck of cards. Most of us eat more than twice the animal proteins we need and most restaurant portions are enough to feed a family. Unless you are an avid body builder, any *excess protein is converted to SUGAR and stored as FAT*. Yes, excess chicken or even salmon can make you FAT! Even worse, many of the animals we consume are fed unhealthy diets full of toxins, antibiotics, and hormones. Those toxins persist and even become concentrated up the food chain. You are only as healthy as the health of whatever you eat.

Look for:

- Meats and dairy from organic, grass-fed animals (grass-fed meats have more anti-inflammatory omega 3 fat while corn-fed meats contain more inflammatory omega 6)
- Organic free-range poultry and eggs
- Wild caught fish
- Make your own or buy organic bone broths shown to particularly support healing and make a good base for super healthy soups, stews, and chili

If eating organic seems too expensive, tally up what you are spending every year on medical costs, or consider the value of staving off disability for a decade. What is one extra quality year of life worth to you? What is the real cost of disease and early disability? You decide whether your long-term health and vitality are worth the investment. As author Elizabeth Gilbert once quoted a mentor,

"What choices are you willing to make, and what will you give up, to have the life you are pretending you want?"

No doubt this module has given you a lot to digest. Pick at least two strategies that you can easily implement TODAY. Enlist your support people to help you. Consider which areas create the biggest opportunity for impact. Just giving up sodas, even diet ones, and juices is a huge commitment for many but I guarantee doing so will save you hundreds if not thousands of dollars annually and decades of misery.

The more healthy habits you adopt, the better but only if you stick with them, even if imperfectly. No turning back now. You are on your way and your commitment is essential.

CHAPTER 1 OPTIMIZING HEALTH SUMMARY

- Commit to stewardship of your health
- Create your environment for success and collaborate with others to support your commitment to health

- Ditch sodas, juices, sugars, fast food and junk food
- If overweight, set a goal to lose at least 10lb prior to surgery
- Boost hydration to half your body weight in total fluid ounces daily
- Boost intake of colorful *organic* fruits and vegetables (at least 3 cups greens, 3 cups colorful veggies daily) and plenty of fiber
- Incorporate healthy fats like high quality extra virgin olive oil, olives, avocado, nuts/seeds into main meals
- Healthy lean protein in small portions (wild-caught fish, organic poultry/eggs/dairy, grass-fed beef, legumes), organic bone broths

Your body is a temple...
but not if you treat it like a garbage dump

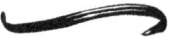

Chapter 2:

Optimizing Detoxification: Prepping The Liver And GI Tract For Surgery

Illustrative Story

The Physician Learns a Lesson – What Doctors Don't Know CAN Hurt You

I was at the "pinnacle" of my career, directing a prestigious Family Medicine Residency and boasting Board Exam scores above the 90th percentile. I knew my stuff, and loved teaching and caring for patients. As many of us do, I also believed I was "pretty healthy." When I needed surgery for a skin cancer on my eyelid and a benign cyst on my wrist, I cavalierly disregarded potential risks and my health status going in. I had blind trust in my surgeon, anesthesiology staff (you rarely get to meet your anesthesiologist ahead of surgery) and my own "pretty good" health. Hence, I plunged into surgery completely unprepared. Unfortunately, the surgery took twice as long as expected and afterward I experienced significant problems with memory, concentration, and focus. I suffered weeks of brain fog and chronic fatigue. My energy was so low that gravity seemed too *heavy. I could barely get off the floor. I also experienced muscle pain typical of a condition called fibromyalgia.*

After this experience, I desperately dove into studying what could be possible root causes of my challenges with colleagues in the field of Functional Medicine. I studied pharmacogenetics and found I was a "poor metabolizer" for many medications and had several genetic issues, or SNPs, that impaired my ability to clear toxins and hormones. I learned too late, that these same genetic findings likely contributed to my Mom's multiple cancers and my sister's premature demise from breast cancer at the devastating age of 42. I studied advanced nutritional testing and found I had dozens of nutrient deficiencies, likely due to my diet full of processed foods, daily diet sodas, and the powerful acid blockers on which I had been dependent on for years. My Functional Medicine physician uncovered hormone and neurochemical imbalances due to insufficient sleep and woefully inadequate stress management strategies.

I started to make small habit changes. Initially eliminating all sodas and adding more plant-based whole foods daily. Next, I eliminated gluten grains, magically evaporating all my muscle and joint pains, acid reflux and digestive issues. I added daily exercise and meditation practice – learning how to breathe effectively for the first time ever. I corrected nutrient deficits, rapidly reviving my energy and focus. I literally remember taking my three small children to the playground the first moment my energy turned on like a light switch. I actually felt like playing with them instead of just lying on the grass while they played. Prioritizing 8 hours of sleep nightly, for the first time in decades, along with the diet changes, stress management, and nutrient support naturally resurrected my hormones, resolving "premature ovarian failure."

I had thought I was healthy before but, in retrospect, I was a walking disaster headed towards a path of early disability, probable cancer, and potential dementia. These minor habit changes gave rise to this phenomenal glow of health and vitality I never knew was possible. Even my telomeres, genetic markers of aging, continue growing longer over the past decades, meaning I am literally getting younger at the genetic level!

Ultimately, I realized that despite all that I had learned and taught through my fifteen-year academic career, I was just beginning to grasp the roots of truly optimal health. In the nearly two decades since I left academic medicine to found LifeScape, I have witnessed hundreds of similar brilliant health transformations. We continue to learn, revise strategies, collaborate with and learn from our patients. The more we learn, the more we realize how little we know. Humbling, yet profoundly liberating. We are each our own clinical trial. Never sell yourself short. We all have FAR more power over our health than we realize, and, as I prophetically stated in my last speech to graduating residents, real solutions rarely come from a prescription pad.

I hope you are already engaged and enjoying mindfully nurturing your body with more healthy plant-based foods as discussed in Chapter 1. What we consume is also essential to supporting our body's ability to clear toxins. Chapter 2 is where we get down and dirty in understanding the science of detoxification, or supporting your body's ability to clear toxins.

No matter how clean our lifestyle, we are absolutely inundated with environmental toxins – chemicals that wreak havoc on our systems, contributing to obesity and diabetes, chronic pain, hormone dysfunction, mood and sleep problems, trigger cancers or autoimmune disorders, and neurologic problems from autism and attention deficit to Alzheimer's and Parkinson's Diseases.

Although our bodies work diligently around the clock to neutralize and clear toxins, our systems are easily overwhelmed. Since the industrial revolution, our environmental exposures include more than one hundred thousand new chemicals with more added every day. Some, such as highly toxic DDT, were banned decades ago yet still show up in people because they are incredibly persistent in the environment, accumulating in the fat of animals at the top of the food chain. Think of that the next time you bite into a juicy prime rib or greasy burger.

Our exposome, or the total exposures we each face throughout a lifetime, includes everything we ingest, the air we breathe, objects we touch or apply topically, even our activities and the psychological stresses we face. Your exposome influences whether your gut microbes are healthy or not, which, in turn, determines whether certain genes get turned on or off, dictating your risk of cancer, mood disorders, obesity and diabetes, autoimmune conditions (where your immune system turns against the body), chronic disease or dementia. The health of your microbiota even determines health risks you pass along to your offspring. Studies revealed an AVERAGE of 200 industrial chemicals and pollutants in umbilical cord blood of newborns in the US – including pesticides and herbicides, consumer product ingredients like chemicals from fast food packaging, BPA from can liners and plastic bottles, phthalates also from plastics and foods, PFOA from Teflon pans, flame retardants, to name just a few. According to the Environmental Working Group, *"Of the 287 chemicals we detected in umbilical cord blood, we know that 180 cause cancer in humans or animals, 217 are toxic to the brain and nervous system, and 208 cause birth defects or abnormal development in animal tests. The dangers of pre- or post-natal exposure to this complex mixture of carcinogens, developmental toxins and neurotoxins have never been studied."*

Some toxins are self-inflicted, including alcohol (a nerve and liver toxin and carcinogen), acetaminophen or Tylenol (a potent liver toxin), smoking or vaping, and the medications and supplements we take. Others permeate our food supply like herbicides and pesticides, are added to skin, dental and haircare products we apply daily, leach from cookware and plastics, or off-gas from carpets, fabrics and furnishings. It might surprise you that the highest food source of toxic arsenic is RICE; the highest levels of glyphosate, or Round-up herbicide, now considered a potential carcinogen by the World

Health Organization and banned by many countries, are in grains, particularly OAT cereals including oatmeal and Cheerios. Kraft Mac & Cheese contains the highest phthalate levels of any food. Sorry kids. Is it any wonder our health has gone haywire?

In addressing detoxification, and your overall health, you must get to know and love your microbiota - the trillions of microorganisms that inhabit our body's every surface, including eyes, ears, nose, respiratory tract, mouth, skin, gastrointestinal and genitourinary tracts. We are just beginning to get a glimpse of the critical supporting role of these microbes, and their genetic activity, or microbiome. Your microbiome impacts whether you are healthy or sick, fat or thin, depressed or happy, inflamed or not. Your microbiome is as crucial as the liver for detoxification, produces hormones and neuro-transmitters influencing mood and brain function, and keeps your immune system on track fighting off infections and cancers without runaway inflammation or autoimmune triggering. Unfortunately, our microbes are increasingly devastated by all the antibiotics we take or feed to animals we consume, and by excessive cleanliness with antibacterial soaps, lotions, toothpastes and mouthwash. Our microbiota cannot survive on our standard phytonutrient and fiber-poor, highly processed, chemically-laden diets. Just 5 days of an antibiotic can disrupt your microbiome for months or years. This is our precious coral reef – a bacterial ecosystem upon which we are absolutely dependent. The health of every ecosystem, from the rain forest to the human microbiome, depends on diversity and balance.

Now be sure to complete your Am I a Good Surgical Candidate Survey (Appendix 1). If you scored 2 or less, you are already a detoxification rock star so keep doing what you are doing. If you scored 3-9, pay close attention to this chapter. If you scored over 10, please pursue extra help. Seek an appointment with our team at LifeScape or a Functional Medicine or Naturopathic provider for more intensive evaluation and medically-supervised detoxification support. I am not talking juice cleanses and fasts here, which can be dangerous in a highly toxic state. Your body locks toxins away in fat to protect you from them, so fasting or rapid weight loss can unload a toxic avalanche. Medical detoxification includes evidence-based biochemical support for both phases of liver detoxification and specific strategies to address toxin clearance through your gut microbiota. Undergoing surgery in a highly toxic state dramatically increases your risks of complications, prolonged hospitalization, and even death. If at all possible, defer surgery as long as it takes to achieve a healthier state.

During surgery, your body may experience a number of stressful insults:

- Stress hormones from anxiety or pain and drugs that stress the system
- Days of inadequate nutrition and potential deficiency of critical nutrients
- Exposure to many new chemicals including antiseptics and anesthetic agents
- Antibiotics and sometimes bowel cleansing which dangerously disrupt your gut microbial balance, increasing the risk for infections and impaired healing

- Narcotic pain medicines that cloud consciousness, eventually increase pain sensitivity, impair gut motility and immune function
- Injury and inflammation from the underlying condition or surgery itself

I do not mention these to scare you but to prepare. As Ben Franklin said, *"By failing to prepare, you are preparing to fail."* We will work to minimize as many challenges as we can.

You can see it is absolutely critical we do everything possible to limit input of toxic exposures and maximize output - our body's ability to neutralize and clear toxins efficiently, at all times but ESPECIALLY as we prepare for surgery.

Strategies to Minimize Toxic Exposures

- SHIFT DIET PLANT-BASED, eating organic as much as possible at least for the "Dirty Dozen" most pesticide-laden foods as discussed in Chapter 1
- KEEP ANIMAL PROTEINS SMALL, (make meat a side dish – grass-fed, wild-caught, organic) minimizing those raised in unhealthy conditions or at the top of the food chain where toxins accumulate
- EAT ORGANIC GRAINS/OATS, unless you relish the thought of a nice bowl of herbicide for breakfast, AVOID genetically-modified foods
- REVIEW strategies to minimize toxin exposures
- REVIEW the list of HIDDEN HAZARDS IN YOUR MEDICINE CABINET (**Appendix 4**) and discontinue all

but essential medications and supplements approved by your medical team to support liver detoxification, critical nutrients for your immune system and healing, and to maintain or restore healthy microbial balance

- AVOID ALCOHOL for at least 2 weeks prior to surgery and until fully healed and completely off all pain medicine. Seek help if you struggle with abstaining
- STOP ASPIRIN, NSAID PAIN RELIEVERS (such as ibuprofen, naproxen, Celebrex, meloxicam, etc), fish oil, and HERBAL PRODUCTS at least 1 week prior to surgery or per your surgeon's instruction
- OPTIMIZING CLEARANCE OF TOXINS: Your body brilliantly clears toxins through multiple pathways. Here are some of the best strategies to support clearance:
  - HYDRATE with at least 60-70 oz of filtered water daily to boost blood flow and clear out toxins through urine, stool, your lymphatic system and sweat
  - Ditch plastics (bottles, storage containers) and never cook in plastic
  - Try a cup or two of organic Dandelion or Matcha green tea daily
  - EAT THE RAINBOW, not the rainbow of artificially colored sports drinks or gelatins, but the rainbow of naturally colorful fruits and vegetables supporting key nutrients you need for detoxification and healing
  - Aim for at least 3 cups of greens, 3 cups of colorful vegetables daily and 2 fruits

- Why no juices? Fiber is one of the healthiest components of fruits and vegetables, especially for detoxification and feeding your microbiome. Stripping the fiber from fruits, creates a sugar bomb. Excess sugar in the system is toxic to ALL tissues, accelerates aging, belly and liver fat accumulation, and slows healing
- BOOST FIBER INTAKE gradually, always with plenty of water, to feed your gut flora and to bind and clear toxins. Aim for at least 25 grams of fiber for women, 30 grams for men (this is DOUBLE what most of us are consuming)
- SWEAT, BRUSH, & SOAK. Skin and lymphatic system are brilliant organs for detoxification so working up a good sweat through exercise, rebounding on a mini-trampoline, or using an infrared sauna can be helpful. Be sure to rinse off sweat immediately to keep toxins from reabsorbing. Soak your feet or bathe in a tub with Epsom salts (you can also add baking soda and a few drops of essential oils like lavender, citrus, or mint). Dry brushing the skin 10 minutes a day or lymphatic massage boost lymphatic flow. These will only work if you are well-hydrated
- Frequently wash linens to avoid re-absorbing toxins through the skin. Preferably use hypoallergenic products free of chemical fragrances or fabric softeners that add a layer of chemicals to linens
- Consider medically supporting detoxification pathways. Our supplement recommendations include

fiber and key nutrients to support all phases of liver detoxification plus probiotics to support optimize gut microbial balance.

Congratulations on making it through the toughest, but MOST IMPORTANT chapter on your journey to assuring you are in the absolutely best shape possible for surgery. This information is not intended to treat any medical condition nor override the recommendations of your medical team. My goal is to support and empower you with a few lifestyle strategies toward achieving the vibrant health you deserve. Keep up the good work and remember even small habit changes have huge impact.

CHAPTER 2
OPTIMIZING DETOXIFICATION SUMMARY

- Avoid alcohol (liver/brain toxin & cancer-promoting) for 2 weeks prior to surgery and until off all pain medicines, muscle relaxants
- Reevaluate your medications with your primary care provider to minimize potentially risky medications
- Get your gut in gear with more fluids, fiber, activity
- Support a healthy microbiome with plant-based, predominantly organic whole-food diet (avoiding refined/processed foods) and by avoiding alcohol and minimizing acid blockers, antibiotics
- Incorporate frequent deep breathing to support clearing toxins via lungs

- Support detoxification through skin and lymphatics with sweating, dry-brushing, foot soaks or baths with Epsom salts
- Incorporate supplements to support liver and GI tract detoxification
- If high toxicity risk (obesity, heavy alcohol intake, chronic narcotic or hormone use or score >10 on the "Am I a Healthy Surgical Candidate" survey), consider intensive work with clinician or nutritionist trained in functional medicine (see **Appendix 8**)

Life is tough but so are you

Chapter 3:

Mentally Preparing For Surgery

Illustrative Story

Best Stressed: To Worry Is to Wish for What You Do Not Want

Chronic anxiety and worry plagued Joan her entire life. A victim of horrific abuse at the hands of her mother, she suffered head injuries and significant physical and emotional trauma throughout her childhood. However, she persevered, eventually enjoying decades happily married to a wonderfully supportive spouse and successfully raising healthy children, breaking the cycle of abuse.

However, anxiety and worry took their toll on Joan physically, resulting in terrifying blood pressure spikes in response to any perceived stressor. The blood pressure spikes, along with other factors that made her blood more prone to clots, resulted in multiple strokes. Fortunately, Joan is a survivor and rebounded from each stroke with remarkably minimal residual symptoms.

When faced with an elective surgical procedure, Joan quickly became overwhelmed with worry and indecision. Blood pressure began spiking again and blood tests revealed signs of inflammation. **Stress***, and the fight, flight, fright response it* *triggers, **is inflammatory**, unless we learn how to control it. She experienced difficulty sleeping and deferred procedures that promised to significantly improve her quality of life.*

I helped Joan lean into the anxiety and worry, observing, accepting, and questioning her perseverating negative thoughts. We both observed how worry and anxiety resulted in a negative mindset, fixating only on everything that could go wrong with the proposed surgery. Someone once said, "To worry is to wish for what you do not want." We tend to get what we focus on and fear is a magnet. We delved deeply into Joan's deepest fears and helped her recognize and question fears that were overblown. Joan was encouraged to work with a clinical psychologist. She was also prescribed several simple homework assignments, including a gratitude journal in which she would write down anything that inspired or uplifted her, touched her heart, or made her laugh each day. She agreed to try deep breathing and a daily walk outdoors. Breathing activates the calming parasympathetic nervous system (the opposite of the adrenalin-fueled, sympathetic or fight, flight, fright nervous system). Joan learned she could bring her blood pressure down 10 points with just 4 deep cleansing breaths a few times daily. Also, nothing boosts mood better than daily exercise. Attention to healthy sleep with a calming bedtime ritual helped her settle anxious thoughts at night.

Although anxiety and worry will always plague Joan, she learned easy and empowering strategies that help her mindfully attend to the negative thoughts, challenge them, and balance them with positive habits of mind. Once her practice was firmly established, she let us know she was ready to have surgery and entered the operating room with a healthy positive mindset and all went smoothly.

These first chapters gave you a lot to digest, literally and figuratively, because what you consume and how you clear toxins is fundamental to your health. No doubt, it can feel overwhelming, especially given the urgency of getting in shape for what is arguably the biggest athletic event of your life. You are in training, and committed to active stewardship of your health to assure you are as fit as humanly possible when you enter the operating room. It is possible to reverse diabetes or severe inflammation in a matter of weeks if you have the right tools, strategies and mindset. Remember to focus on a few key actions that are likely to be the most impactful for you. Small steps, like just eliminating added sugars and refined grains or eating more fresh fruits and vegetables daily can have massive impact over time.

My health dramatically transformed and I feel decades younger since I began learning functional medicine and understanding the impact of my daily lifestyle choices on my physiology. I began taking small definitive action steps like giving up sodas, breaking my toxic daily Diet Coke habit (I swear there is something addictive in their secret formula). Diet Coke wreaked havoc on my sleep, mood (aspartame is a *neuroexcitotoxin* or chemical that can aggravate stress, anxiety, and headaches), and metabolism (artificial sugars increase diabetes risk as much or more than sugar.) Later, I experimented with giving up gluten grains and found they were causing my chronic joint and muscle pain, stiffness, reflux, gas and bloating. Finally, I committed, with great difficulty, to developing a daily meditation habit and prioritizing sleep to boost my mood and stress tolerance. I had always thought I had no time for activities I saw as nonproductive but eventually saw the benefits in terms of improved focus, productivity, energy, vitality, and mood. I credit sleep and meditation with my business success and literally getting younger in every way.

Over time, I shifted my diet more organic and plant-based, reduced chemicals used in our home, and committed to getting active every day. My telomeres, genetic markers of aging that normally shorten with age, have progressively lengthened, eventually equivalent to a 25-year-old at 58! I am literally getting younger at the genetic level. My evolution occurred over 15 years and I am asking you to transform in a few weeks. I applaud your willingness to dive in and do your best in a cram course. However, please do not be too hard on yourself. *Perfection is not the goal.* If you slip, just take a breath of gratitude for your health, remember *why* this commitment is so important to you, and get back at it. A life of deprivation is not a life. You can incorporate occasional treats and things you love as long as treats are supported on a foundation of at least 75% healthy intake. Pay attention to how you feel when you overindulge versus when you eat clean. My hope is that several of the habits learned in this program stick, becoming your roadmap for a more vibrant and fulfilling life.

In Chapter 3, we address the Mind-Body connection. How we think, perceive and manage stress, and recharge is every bit as important to our health as diet and exercise. As every athlete knows, mental fitness is an essential part of preparation. As Coach Bobby Knight said, *"The will to succeed is important but what's more important is the will to prepare."* In preparing for surgery, we want to set a positive intention and mindset, learn positive stress-moderating strategies, and learn how to face and channel anxiety and worry in healthy ways.

Stress gets a bad rap – we hear so much negativity about it. However, stress actually primes us to grow, adapt, perform at our best and heal. Stress itself is not lethal, but how we choose to handle it can be. I've cared for Holocaust survivors who endured the depths of inhumanity, people who endured brutality for years as prisoners of war, accident and burn victims or those with severed spines, lost limbs or excruciating pain, and many others who have endured unimaginable losses. They taught me that those who thrive in the midst of the unimaginable are those who seek joy in every moment and indulge in gratefulness for every tiny blessing. Their recipe for resilience:

HAPPINESS is a VERB
ATTITUDE is a CHOICE
GRATEFULNESS is your ACTION PLAN

MENTAL PREPARATION STRATEGIES

The first and most critical step in mentally preparing for any major challenge is:

SET YOUR INTENTION

Intention is a bit like setting a course with a compass, then mapping the steps to move toward your destination. Define your goal clearly: For example, your goal might be: "I will breeze through surgery without complications, heal quickly and easily." Then define what steps will you take toward your goal today such as, "I will eat a large colorful salad and a healthy smoothie today and walk for at least 30 minutes." Using a daily habit checklist helps clarify and solidify your intention by reviewing your ultimate goal, your WHY or crucial reasons that goal is so important for you, and your daily action steps to move you toward your goal. A goal without an action plan is a wish, not a goal. The more actively and repeatedly you visualize achieving your ultimate goal, and experience what that achievement will feel like, the more solid and achievable your intention becomes.

The next step in priming your mindset is:

OBSERVE SELF-TALK

Our brains are a relentless producer of thoughts. Is your constant machine gun fire of brain chatter positive, encouraging, and inspiring, or is it negative, demeaning, and full of worry or hopelessness? As one patient commented, *"if anyone spoke to my kids or me the way I speak to myself, I'd pummel them!"* Humans are hard-wired to focus on negative inputs. Attending to threats is our evolutionary survival programming that helped us avoid danger. However, with daily practice, we can learn to recognize our automatic negative thoughts (or ANTs) and tame them or replace them with more productive thoughts. Adopting mindfully positive self-talk also takes daily practice. I am constantly on the alert for my own toxic thinking, noticing thoughts like "I'm terrible at this," "I hate technology," "I've never been disciplined" or phrases of lax commitment, "I might...," "I'll try...," I hope to...," "I wish...," I should..." or "I can't..." Bulletproof Founder and biohacker Dave Aspery aptly terms these phrases "weasel words."

What are your ANTs and Weasel Words? Pay attention, catch them, accept them and try to immediately replace them when they inevitably arise.

The next step in mental preparation:

LEAN INTO ANXIETY AND WORRY

Someone once said, *"To worry is to pray for what you do not want."*

Anxiety is the rumination about what might happen in the future or our perception of what occurred in the past. Unfortunately, our pill-for-an-ill culture encourages us to pop a pill for every negative sensation (pain, anxiousness, worry, sadness, irritability.) Hence, thousands are losing their lives to addiction, overdose, alcohol abuse, and suicide. When you numb the bad, you numb the good as well.

Anxiety and worry are simply thoughts.

Thoughts might carry important messages we need to heed or thoughts might overly catastrophize risks and snowball into an avalanche of useless, joy-stealing worry. The antidote to anxious worry is to center yourself in THIS MOMENT, focus on your breath, and watch mindfully as your anxious thoughts pass by like clouds in the sky. Examine them with wonder, asking yourself, "is there something here I need to reevaluate, and do I need to change course?" Another option is to lean into anxiety, peering deeper, asking "Is that really true?" "Could there be another explanation?" "How would I feel if that were not true?"

If you are prone to catastrophic thinking, runaway anxiety, or are inundated by ANTs (automatic negative thoughts), I encourage you to check out:

- Any of the amazing meditation and mindfulness apps available
- Tapping, an emotional freedom technique available at tapping.com
- Local or online courses on mindfulness and meditation
- Any of John Kabat Zinn's books on mindfulness
- Journaling
- Restorative exercise like yoga, pilates, dance or tai chi
- Biofeedback tools such as HeartMath or Muse
- Devices to activate the vagus nerve (parasympathetic/calming nervous system)
- Seeking professional help from a therapist or physician

Getting professional help is critical if your anxiety or worry significantly impair your relationships or ability to function. My favorite prescription for anyone mired in negativity comes from Mind-Body Psychologist Dr. Joan Borysenko:

> "Every day, look for something that:
> inspired you,
> made you laugh, and
> touched your heart;
> Shifting your focus towards the positive
> immediately shifts your experience"

JUST BREATHE

Your breath is an ever-present pressure release valve, allowing you to activate your calming nervous system; controlling blood pressure, heart rate, and stress hormones, reducing pain and relaxing tense muscles. It is FREE, always readily available, and carries no addictive potential. Any woman who used Lamaze breathing methods during childbirth knows the power of this amazing tool. Those who practice regular breathing techniques through meditation can sometimes induce a hypnotic trance and even undergo surgery using only the power of meditation for anesthesia. I am certainly not suggesting you forgo anesthesia, but that intensive meditation practice could reduce the amount of anesthesia or pain medication needed and expedite clearance of those medications.

Create a mini deep breathing habit by tying a couple deep breaths to something you already do several times a day – like booting up your computer, washing your hands, starting your car, or waiting at a stop light. Try always to breathe slowly through your nose. My mini-habit is to take a deep breath whenever I tell a patient to and every time I wash my hands (20 seconds of hand-washing equals about 3 deep breaths). Learn and practice deep breathing techniques (breathe counting in for 4, hold for 7, and out for 8) several times per day, or use a breathing program on your iPhone, Fitbit, or meditation app to remind and guide you.

FILTER YOUR INPUTS

Toxic inputs pollute our mindsets. Consider how much of what you read, watch, listen to or discuss with others is negative or full of anger, blame, shame, criticism, or complaint. What do you focus on or share on social media? Fortunately, although we all are victim to mind-control from many forces, we have complete control to CHOOSE our inputs. We can quite easily break the negativity habit by choosing to read, watch, listen to, follow, or share inspiring, empowering, encouraging messaging. We also choose the people with whom we congregate. Dose yourself liberally with "life-infusing" people and scale back contact with "life-o-suction" or "energy vampires," those spewing toxic shame, blame, criticism or complaint. Before getting too judgmental, we all need to look in the mirror. How often are we showing up as life infusion people? I guarantee, the more you focus on inspiring, empowering, and encouraging others, the more you will receive the same in return. As we taught our children, life is like a swing-set, what you put out there comes right back at you.

Last, but not least:

RECHARGE WITH HEALTHY SLEEP

Healthy sleep is one of the most critical yet often neglected pillars of our health. Most of us are not getting close to the 7-8 hours necessary nightly for optimal functioning. We now understand that, during sleep, the brain clears out toxic waste and stores memories. Studies have documented that at every age the protein markers of Alzheimer's dementia are present in the spinal fluid of subjects after REM sleep disruption on just one night. Sleep is critical to optimal hormone balance, blood sugar control, immune system function, and virtually every system in the body. Carving just 30 minutes a day off of healthy sleep increases stress hormone cortisol levels. Excess cortisol, in turn, elevates blood sugar and insulin, results in belly and liver fat accumulation, and reduces the production of testosterone and estrogens. Contrary to all the advertisements, "low T" does not mean you need a life-long drug, but usually that you are suffering from deficient sleep, stress management, and nutrition. Drugged sleep, whether through alcohol or any other sleep medicine, including over-the-counter ones, is NOT healthy sleep. Alcohol is particularly toxic to deep restorative sleep.

Critical steps to healthy sleep:

- Taper off or significantly minimize caffeine, and consume none after noon
- Minimize or eliminate alcohol – avoiding any within 3 hours of bedtime
- Eat a light dinner, fasting completely for 3 hours before bedtime
- Hydrate with lots of filtered water, especially if you have vascular disease
- Unplug from electronics 90 minutes before bed
- Eliminate electronics from your bedroom and time out Wi-Fi overnight
- Engage in a soothing nighttime ritual
- Set your next day to-do list priorities (offload your brain) and tuck it away
- Keep the bedroom cool and completely dark or wear an eye mask
- Journal/meditate/pray on gratitude or your daily wins
- Cuddle time with partner, kids, or pet
- Relaxing bath with Epsom salts and lavender oil
- Use relaxing essential oils in a diffuser or spray on your pillow
- Read something calming or uplifting
- Keep the bedroom cool, optimally 65 degrees, for sleep

CHAPTER 3
MENTALLY PREPARING SUMMARY

- Manage stress with daily habits (prayer, meditation, gratitude, deep breathing)
- Set your intention daily
- Observe self-talk noticing and gently reframing automatic negative thoughts (ANTS) and "weasel words" of flimsy commitment
- Lean into anxiety and learn to observe emotions and allow them to pass
- Learn and practice deep breathing techniques (breathe in for 4, hold for 7, out for 8) several times per day or use breathing program on phones, Fitbits or similar devices, or meditation apps
- Filter negative inputs and maximize inputs that inspire, empower, and encourage you or make you laugh
- Indulge in healthy sleep

Control is an illusion...
all we control is how well we prepare &
how we steer when we hit the rapids

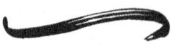

Chapter 4:

Reducing Complications After Surgery

Illustrative story

Best-Laid Plans Failed to Avert a Snowball of Complications

A straightforward joint replacement turned into a nightmare for Elaine. Elaine was the perfectly compliant patient every surgeon loves. She had been through surgery before and did everything asked of her. Surgery itself went smoothly, although she was slow to recover from anesthesia, a clue that her body's detoxification processes were not ideal.

Elaine appropriately received narcotic pain medications after this major orthopedic surgery. As is often the case, she suffered severe constipation from them. The narcotics so significantly shut down her digestive motility, that she developed intractable vomiting, dehydration, and electrolyte imbalances, necessitating readmission to the hospital. While hospitalized she was bedridden, unable to walk very often and developed a blood clot in addition to a urinary tract infection. The blood clot fortunately did not travel to the lungs (where it would have caused a pulmonary embolism, which could have been lethal), but required Elaine to take blood thinners for several months. Antibiotics given for the urinary infection then resulted in c. difficile colitis – a very severe and sometimes lethal diarrheal illness that can be very challenging to cure.

Elaine's experience illustrates how easily one minor medication side effect can snowball into a litany of extremely high risk, potentially lethal complications. The toll on her was significant, two additional weeks in the hospital, hospital bills in the tens of thousands of dollars, weeks on expensive antibiotics and months on blood thinners, and the emotional toll that has her dreading any potential future surgery. I have known patients who have died or lost loved ones from blood clot complications or require removal of the colon and lifetime with a colostomy bag from c. difficile colitis. Anticipatory strategies can avert most of these complications.

Completely avoidable catastrophes witnessed over the years prompted me to develop this course. I lost a loved one due to inadequate preoperative screening, lung complications and adverse medication reactions that resulted in six grueling months in the hospital before he needlessly succumbed. I watched helplessly as family, friends and patients endured horrific complications, protracted hospitalizations, or readmissions that were potentially deadly and completely avoidable. The costs—physical, mental, and financial—inflict a huge toll on patients and their families, their surgeons, and even their primary care providers! Catastrophic medical expenses are the number one reason behind most bankruptcies in the United States. I hope to prevent many more financial and medical casualties.

However, should we choose to accept it, we have more control than we think over our health outcomes. Choosing to be active warriors rather than passive victims makes all the difference. Most post-surgical complications, and even deaths, are avoidable by understanding the risks and proactively engaging in simple preventive strategies before and after surgery. The better you understand the possible risks, the more rapidly you or your health advocate can alert your medical team if warning signs of a problem arise. Rapid action can be life-saving.

Health advocates are worth considering. Hospitals are very confusing and busy systems with overtaxed staff rotating constantly. The lack of continuity means no single caregiver really knows you well. After surgery, you may be temporarily incapable of advocating for yourself, so I encourage engagement with a knowledgeable health advocate who can ask questions, oversee progress, and make sure you get the attention you need promptly. An advocate could be a medically astute family member or friend, caregiver, your own primary care physician, or you can hire a professional nurse advocate. It is important that your advocate know the details of your health status, especially important information about medication intolerances or preferences, family history which gives us clues to your potential risks, and your active medical issues and recent test results. The best advocates are excellent diplomats, working respectfully and collaboratively with your medical team, without being adversarial. Being overbearing, rude, or critical towards your care team is rarely in anyone's best interest. Healthcare providers are all hard-working, caring people doing their best for their patients, often under trying conditions. Although none of us is perfect, and we all have days when we are not at our best, it is always best to presume health care professionals are well-intentioned.

Your surgical team will review potential risks with you, but by educating yourself you become your own best advocate. In the online Preparing for Surgery program (www.optimizesurgery.com), we delve deeper into potential risks, providing specific steps to mitigate or prevent them, or at least recognize when immediate action is necessary.

Appendix 5 outlines a comprehensive list of complications and strategies developed by our team of medical professionals. It combines years of experience into one convenient guide covering many of the most common complications to be aware of after surgery and best steps you can take to prepare.

Although it might seem scary, I encourage you to take time to review this list, share it with your advocates, and create your own personalized action plan of preventive strategies. These strategies again represent some of the best approaches our research has proven to help facilitate a fast recovery. Strategies include recommended diet, nutritional, fitness, and mental wellness plans. As Ben Franklin stated, "An ounce of prevention is worth a pound of cure."

CHAPTER 4
REDUCING COMPLICATIONS SUMMARY

- Assign a health advocate who can support you before/after surgery
- Work with your advocate to learn the potential surgical complications and strategies to minimize your risk
- Review signs and symptoms that require you to seek help immediately
- Make a plan to maintain a clean plant-based diet rich in nutrients that support healing, stay well hydrated, and remain active after surgery

Your body's ability to heal is greater than anyone has permitted you to believe

Chapter 5:

Musculoskeletal Fitness For Surgery: Assuring Healthy Muscles, Bones, Tendons And Joints

Illustrative Story

Proactive Training for Surgery

Gary realized his health had gradually deteriorated from benign neglect. He enjoyed indulging in delicious food and wine, skimping on exercise and sleep, gradually gaining weight and progressively suffering disability from degenerative joint disease (osteoarthritis).

He had diligently gotten his annual "check-up," where his doctors had repeatedly suggested that he "lose a few pounds" and prescribed him several medications for emerging chronic conditions including arthritis and high blood pressure (hypertension), as well as potent acid-blockers for acid reflux. Gary, a bright executive, knew a little about the potential risks and side effects from those medications. However, when faced with the prospect of replacing both his knees, Gary realized he needed a more proactive, transformative approach to his health.

He recognized that the pill-for-an-ill strategy was causing him to accumulate a list of daily prescriptions while his health kept declining.

Gary appreciated health was his most critical asset. He astutely invested in working with a physician certified in Functional Medicine, who led a team including a Functional Medicine-certified Nutritionist / Health Coach and a Fitness Trainer. Advanced assessments uncovered multiple root causes of Gary's health issues, including nutrient deficiencies, an inflammatory diet, detoxification risks, muscle weakness and inadequate sleep and stress management resulting in hormone deficiency. Gary worked collaboratively with his team, cleaning up his diet, losing over 10lb in a few weeks, learning how to strengthen the support of his injured joints. The force on your knees is equivalent to 1.5 times your body weight, and even more when walking on an incline. So just a nominal ten-pound weight loss, combined with an anti-inflammatory diet and strengthening the supportive muscles around the joints, can rapidly and dramatically reduce disability. He learned to prioritize sleep and incorporated some simple stress management mini-habits. He was able to wean off acid-blockers, dangerous NSAID anti-inflammatory medicines, and even his blood pressure medicine.

Not only was Gary able to cruise through a double knee replacement and recover at a pace astounding to his surgical team, he enjoyed renewed energy and vitality that has persisted more than a year later. Although some of his habits, like the joy of rich food and wine, have resurfaced, he understands the importance of maintaining moderation and healthy balance.

Musculoskeletal fitness is key to physical and mental health. Consider the concept of disability, or the loss of an aspect of your motor function. Disability often sneaks up on us almost imperceptibly. A few years ago, I realized I was struggling to lift my carry-on suitcase into an overhead rack on an airplane. I secretly hoped they would gate-check my bag so I could avoid this embarrassing ritual. That lack of ability is *disability*. Fortunately, I paid attention to the wake-up call, took action and started weight training. Now I can easily heft my own bag and help others with theirs. Some struggle to rise from the floor or even up from a chair or toilet seat. None of us wish to become disabled, yet **Americans spend more years in chronic disease and disability than those in any other economically advanced nation**. However, we hold the keys to our own shackles through our daily lifestyle choices. One of my mentors, Dr. Peter Attia, describes the proactive concept of training for your "centenarian Olympics." Visualize and clearly note what you wish to be able to do at 100, then reverse engineer a strategic plan to assure you get there. For example, I would like to be able to lift and hug my great-grandchildren, so I do 20-minute strength-training sessions twice a week and 5 minute mini-sessions daily. One of my 90+ year-old patients does 20 sit-stands from a chair twice a day, determined never to need help rising from a chair or commode.

Our bodies require abundant and diverse movement every bit as critically as we need sleep and nutrition to thrive. When patients ask me, "why does this hurt?" I usually think of what a brilliant miracle it is that the body works as well as it does, given the regular abuse and neglect it endures. Stuffing our feet into restrictive shoes—particularly torturous high heels designed for Barbie Doll feet—and stuffing our rear ends in chairs for hours on end clearly causes real harm. Prolonged sitting confers health risks equivalent to smoking, increasing your risk of bone loss, fractures, arthritis, obesity, diabetes, heart disease and strokes, memory issues, certain cancers, and even mental health problems. Furthermore, just as you cannot truly "catch up" on missed sleep by sleeping in on weekends, you cannot make up for hours of nonstop sitting. Research suggests you need 60–75 minutes per day of moderate-intensity activity to combat the dangers of excessive sitting. On the other end of the fitness spectrum, however, some of us overdose on fitness activities or focus on one type of movement exclusively. Endurance exercise can be great, but has the potential to cause harmful inflammation and even heart injury (studies show a high percentage of men and women completing a marathon have elevated troponin levels – a chemical indicating heart damage). Endurance athletes also risk overuse injury, elevated stress hormones, and depleted gonadal hormones such as testosterone. Doing nothing but running is equivalent to eating a diet of only protein. Moderation and variety are the keys to healthy movement.

Movement is essential to pump blood and lymphatic fluid through the body, through all your organs and your brain, and to clear toxins out via the kidneys, skin and digestive tract. Your digestive tract gets sluggish without movement and skin becomes dull and sallow. Just the impact of your feet on the ground is critical to your brain's blood flow.

Bones only build if stressed, so if you are not stressing the bones every day with impactful exercise, they rapidly deteriorate, regardless of your intake of vitamins or minerals such as vitamin D or calcium. Just 2 minutes of jumping exercise daily can build healthy bone density in the legs and spine. If injured, work with a physical therapist or athletic trainer to exercise around your injury, maintaining fitness rather than letting the rest of the body deteriorate. I remind my patients of quadriplegics who manage to exercise; If they can do it, surely we too can work around less catastrophic injuries, nurturing our bodies with healthy movement.

Muscles support your bones and joints; if allowed to weaken by disuse, your joints become increasingly unstable and prone to injury. If you need surgery for an orthopedic problem, be sure to work with a physical therapist or trainer to build the strength of the muscles around that joint. Surgery repairs a specific localized problem, but the work of rehabilitation requires a holistic approach including nutrition, detoxification, and whole-body movement.

Please attend to the fascia, the thin layer of connective tissue that covers all our muscles like a nylon stocking. Fascia runs from the bottom of your feet to the scalp, incorporating nerves and lymphatic channels. Think of fascia as the human body's internet. Tight, torn, inflamed, or constricted fascia can cause significant mechanical dysfunction in your joints or spine. I suffered 30 years of neck pain from an injury that was resolved with a single myofascial visit over a decade ago. I call my myofascial therapist my "body-whisperer" (see sterlingstructuraltherapy.com for more information). Fascial imbalances are amenable to stretching, myofascial therapy, massage, or roller therapy—if we take care not to traumatize the fascia with overly aggressive techniques.

Another key to musculoskeletal health is posture. Check out your posture by having someone take a picture of you from the side or doing a fit3D or similar assessment. If you find that your palms face backwards when you are standing straight, pay attention. The rounded shoulders and forward shifted head characteristic of those of us constantly glued to our cell phones and computers restrict your lung capacity and put tremendous mechanical stresses on the back, neck, and pelvis.

Excess weight adds significant surgical risk and can hamper recovery. If you are overweight or obese, or your waist circumference is greater than your hip circumference (indicating dangerous metabolic dysfunction), you are metabolically unhealthy and likely have impaired detoxification and immune function. Work aggressively with a nutritionist on achieving a healthier weight prior to elective surgery. Even a loss of just 10% of your bodyweight if overweight or obese dramatically reduces blood sugar and metabolic risks, blood pressure, and the risk of dying prematurely. Carrying just 10 extra pounds of weight causes the lower spine to pull forward, risking pinched nerves or sciatica, and adds hundreds of pounds of pressure on your hips, knees, ankles and feet with every step.

Here are a few Key Daily Moves for a Healthy Body. These movements are simple, safe, can be done at home or work, take minimal time, and require no equipment or special clothing:

Posture – open the chest, as if a string were pulling your sternum, activate your core by sucking in your stomach (most of us can gain 2-3 inches in height just by activating our core) and relax your shoulder blades. Tuck your chin and treat your cellphone neck to frequent isometric stretches against your hands or the headrest in your car.

Flexibility – stand upright or lay on the floor stretching the arms up far overhead, feeling the stretch throughout your torso. Perform chair stretches for upper/lower body by taking turns hugging each knee across your chest to stretch those tight gluteal muscles.

Strength – squats or wall sits are great lower body exercises. Planks are a safe and effective whole-body core and upper body exercise. You can supplement with resistance bands or light weights or wrist/ankle weights to work other muscles.

Balance- just standing on one foot while reading or simple yoga balance poses retrain your balance senses. Yoga, pilates, tai chi, and dance are wonderful for restorative whole-body movements proven to improve balance and mindful breathing and can all be done at your own pace.

Cardio – 15 minutes of high intensity interval training (short bursts of full out cardio alternating with a couple minutes of slower steady activity) or 30 minutes of walking and at least 2 minutes of jumping daily– jumping jacks, jump rope, or jumping on a rebounder (mini-trampoline) all work. However, even just getting up for a few minutes every hour has tremendous benefit. Consider a 78-year-old couple I treated who were in for their 2-hour physicals. They both diligently got up to pace as their phone alarms reminded them to do every hour. Both reliably hit 20,000 steps per day… inspiring role models in training for their centenarian Olympics.

Better yet, get out and play! Sports are a great way to have fun, engage socially and move.

So what are your ideas to move more daily? In the profound words of Nike:

"Just do it"

It is a shame for a man to grow old without seeing the beauty and strength of which his body is capable

Socrates

Chapter 6:

Optimizing Recovery: Clear Toxins, Control Pain, Boost Healing & Promote Immune Function

Illustrative Story

Same Surgery, Two Approaches:
The Road Less Travelled Made All the Difference

Unfortunately, the first bladder repair surgery only helped for about ten years before the urinary incontinence symptoms recurred. Judy had no major issues with the initial procedure and recovered at the expected rate; she needed narcotic pain medications for only a few weeks and was able to drive and get back to most normal activities in a month. However, she was not crazy about having to undergo another surgery, so this time she decided to train for it. She believed in being proactive about her health and took to heart advice that she could influence her outcome.

She enrolled in Preparing for Surgery online (optimizesurgery. com) and committed to changing habits that had been failing her. She had to overcome an addiction to sweets, and found that cutting them out altogether worked better for her than trying to limit herself. She created her own healthy snacks and completely overhauled her pantry and workplace so that only healthy options were available. She traded her nightly cocktail for either a lighter wine spritzer or kombucha (a probiotic drink) in a wine glass as her evening treat. She got moving with fun dance exercise classes and pilates, gaining fun social connections as well as learning healthy, relaxing movement.

Judy lost 15 pounds over 5 weeks before her surgery, went into the procedure feeling healthier than she had in over a decade. She cruised through surgery without any difficulty. The speed of her recovery stunned both Judy and her surgeon. Usually second surgeries involve more scarring, higher risk of complications, and longer recovery. This time, however—likely due to her preparation—she needed narcotic pain medications for only a few days as opposed to a few weeks. She was back to normal activities within 2 weeks, versus a month following the initial surgery. Not only that, a year after her procedure Judy was able to travel to Peru and climb Machu Picchu, a feat she could never have attempted in her previous "pretty healthy" condition. Not only that, she boasted that twenty year olds on the trail could not keep up with her at 68! She is constantly amazed at her restored energy and vitality and notes, "I thought I was healthy but I really had NO IDEA what healthy could be." Never sell yourself short.

Congratulations for sticking with this program. You have made it to the final chapter, have almost certainly begun taking control of your health, and hopefully are already experiencing the benefits in terms of improved vitality or resolving symptoms.

However, if you continue to struggle with even the smallest daily habit changes, PLEASE schedule an appointment with our nutritionist/health coaches or seek similar resources near you to support you through the slow and steady process of learning to heal yourself. Remember, small habit changes, consistently deployed over time, lead to massive impact.

To paraphrase Warren Buffet, the first step in getting out of any hole is to *QUIT DIGGING*. Understand that your health may have taken decades to reach its present state of disrepair, and a few weeks of "good behavior" will not magically resolve everything. In fact, if you are in a really toxic or inflamed state, you could feel worse as you shed decades of abuse and neglect before feeling better. My friend Hayley Cloud, of Living Raw by Grace, tells her inspiring story of health transformation, having healed decades of chronic asthma, rashes, obesity and progressive blindness with a raw vegan diet. She explains how the healing process included a painful period of worsened symptoms. She now glows with incredible health. Push through it. The rewards are worth a bit of pain and discipline.

I remain constantly amazed by the power of the human spirit and the miraculous healing power of the human body when we provide it with the right fuel and TLC, so keep up the GREAT WORK!

As we embark on this last chapter, continue to work through your Daily Habit checklist so you have a daily road map of health optimization priorities on which to focus.

Questions to Ask Your Surgical Team:

Question 1: Will surgery be performed in a hospital (inpatient facility) or ambulatory surgery center (outpatient) and what are that facility's infection control measures?

Question 2: Is any hospitalization or inpatient rehabilitation anticipated after surgery? If so, what is the expected length of stay?

Question 3: What is your expected functional ability when you get home? How quickly can you expect to recover the ability to perform activities of daily living, including walking without assistance, personal hygiene (bathing/showering/toilet use), dressing, driving, shopping, preparing meals, returning to exercise, and returning to work?

Question 4: How long should you expect to need narcotic pain medications or any medicines that might interfere with your ability to think clearly or operate a motor vehicle? What alternatives to narcotic pain medicines does your surgeon suggest?

Question 5: What special care and support needs should you plan for after surgery? What equipment, supplies, or medications should you order in advance?

Question 6: What are the instructions for stopping/starting daily medications and supplements around surgery?

Question 7: Does your insurance cover the facility in which your surgeon operates, the surgical team, and the anesthesiologist? What are the maximal out of pocket expenses you can expect to incur?

Outpatient surgery in an ambulatory surgery center (ASC) is safe and reasonable for many, and is sometimes less expensive and poses reduced risk of exposure to hospital-acquired infections. However, ASCs may not be staffed or outfitted to handle significant complications or emergencies. Transporting an unstable patient with a complication could be risky. Therefore, your surgeon is likely to recommend surgery in a hospital setting for those who:

- Will be undergoing a high-risk procedure
- Are over 65 or frail at any age
- Are overweight or obese
- Have chronic lung disease
- Have high blood pressure or heart rhythm disorders
- Have had any cardiovascular intervention (stents, bypass, valve repair)
- Are at high risk for heart attack or stroke
- Have diabetes or unstable blood sugar
- Are at high risk for blood clots or bleeding complications

- Have an impaired or suppressed immune system
- Have a history of complications with past surgeries

While Disneyland is supposedly the happiest place on earth, hospitals may be the most daunting. The U.S. Centers for Disease Control noted that one in twenty-five hospitalized patients in 2014 developed a hospital-acquired infection. The good news is that most hospitals take infection risk very seriously and many deploy innovative strategies including coating medical equipment with "self-disinfecting" surfaces or employing automated decontamination technologies that use vaporized hydrogen peroxide or UVC light emission to destroy dangerous microbes. Decontamination efforts have intensified with the Covid19 pandemic. Many organizations oversee the safety of hospitals in the United States. Check your hospital's safety grade:

https://www.hospitalsafetygrade.org/

In any inpatient setting, there are several potential challenges to consider:

Ensure Quality Nutrition: While some hospitals now offer nutritious whole, organic foods, many still hire food services that provide low cost, highly processed meals for patients and employees. When sick or injured, and especially when recovering from surgery, your body desperately needs healthful, plant-based whole foods more than ever. With all we know about nutrition today, there is no excuse for serving our sickest patients sweetened and artificially colored juices, electrolyte drinks, gelatins, puddings, fruit juice, soda, canned foods, refined or processed foods, or salty broths. Find out if your hospital offers fresh organic foods and meals. If not, arrange to have food delivered or have friends or family bring healthy alternatives for you. Even one organic fruit and veggie-full smoothie, soup or bowl a day is powerful medicine.

Minimize Infection Risk: Make sure staff and your visitors wash their hands for 20 seconds before and after visiting, use hand-sanitizer, and wear appropriate gloves and/or gowns to prevent contamination. Make sure you understand why any invasive intervention (IV line, catheter, drains, etc) is needed and for how long. You want lines and catheters out as quickly as possible to minimize the risk of serious infections.

Anticipate need for blood: If your surgery might involve significant blood loss, ask your surgeon about "autologous blood donation" – donating a little of your own blood well in advance of surgery to minimize the risk of receiving infected blood.

Limit exposure to chemicals: When possible, drink only filtered water – bring your own stainless or glass water bottle and make sure it is thoroughly washed daily. Question anything applied to your skin. Clearly communicate any allergies, especially to common items like latex gloves or cleaning agents, iodine or betadine, soaps, lotions, or detergents.

Minimize Radiation Exposure: Confirm that any X-rays or CT scans are necessary. Keep track of every procedure done and specialist seen to cross-reference against hospital charges.

Reduce Stress: Ask your nursing staff, if possible, to adjust their monitoring schedules to minimize sleep disruption. Also, ask that they keep the room as dark and quiet as possible for sleep. Bring a sleep mask and ear plugs to avoid rude awakenings from lights and alarms.

Avoid Prolonged Immobility: Even while bed-bound, make sure you sit up and move your body as much as you comfortably can.

Limit Fall Risk: Medications and surgery can result in temporary lightheadedness, weakness, or difficulty with gait and balance. Make sure to wear slip-proof booties or slippers, always follow staff instructions and stand or ambulate only with proper support. If struggling with balance, ask for physical therapy to help you regain strength and fit you for temporary assistive devices like canes or walkers.

Regardless of where you undergo surgery, the goal is to optimize healing and prevent complications. Immune function, healing injured tissues, and clearing toxins require good fluid intake and a healthy diet with sufficient protein, plant-based phytonutrients, vitamins, and minerals. As discussed previously, healthy movement is critical for preventing many complications, including pneumonia and blood clots, promotes gut motility, and supports controlling pain. Continue these important strategies after surgery and make sure your caregivers also review this list.

Post-Op Recovery Check List:

- Drink plenty of filtered water daily
- Continue fiber, adding stool softeners or laxatives if needed, to prevent constipation and keep the colon moving optimally
- Gently resume eating with small portions of easy-to-digest, nutrient dense, organic smoothies or purees, broths and soups, low-sugar yogurt or kefir, herbal teas, or green drinks/vegetable juices
- Remain sitting up for at least 30-60 min after each meal to prevent reflux (food from the stomach washing back up the esophagus) and aspiration into your lungs
- Drink a little caffeine via organic coffee or Dandelion/green/white tea in the morning to help your kidneys clear retained fluid after surgery
- Continue support nutrients for at least 1 month post-op or until fully healed and off narcotic pain medications
- If you receive antibiotics around surgery, certain probiotics, especially the yeast Sacchromyces boulardii and bacteria Lactobacillus acidophilus, L. rhamnosus, and L. casei, have some evidence for preventing antibiotic-associated diarrhea (also known as C. Difficile colitis).
- Consider a Bromelain supplement and the homeopathic oral and/or topical remedy Arnica to support resolution of bruising

- Continue deep breathing exercises at least hourly while awake (this is critical in the first few days after surgery to prevent pneumonia). Splint any painful part with a pillow or your hand to allow for full deep breaths
- Engage throughout each day in stress relieving strategies – deep breathing, music, videos, prayer, meditation, mindfulness, inspirational reading, or journaling
- When cleared to do so, sit up in a chair, stand, and walk as much as possible
- When resting, stretch your whole body (splinting any painful or injured parts): Move your arms and legs, circling hands and feet, and pump your calves at least once an hour while awake to support blood and lymphatic flow. Request venous sequential compression devices (inflatable cuffs that help support sluggish veins and move blood back towards the heart) if likely to be bed-bound for more than a day
- Bathe or soak feet in warm water with Epsom salts to support clearing toxins through your skin
- Until you can shower or bathe, wash your skin off frequently with clean washcloth, gentle soap and water
- After a sponge bath or shower, massage skin with natural oils such as cold-pressed unrefined coconut oil or extra virgin olive oil. Avocado oil, shea butter, grapeseed or jojoba oil are also good options but careful as oils can make surfaces and feet very slippery

- Consider dry brushing or lymphatic massage to support lymphatic flow, but never dry brush thin, fragile or injured skin
- Wear slip-proof slippers or booties to prevent slipping and falling
- Make sure your sheets are changed frequently if not daily in the first few weeks as you sweat out chemicals from anesthetics and antiseptics used during your surgery.
- For help controlling pain, take medications as directed, initially scheduled on a routine basis to stay ahead of the pain
    o Never combine narcotic pain medications with other sedating medicines, including sleeping pills, benzodiazepine anxiety medicines, or alcohol. Sleep apnea must be treated before use of any of sedating medicines or narcotics
    o Consider use of a TENs unit, guided imagery or meditation, or trial of acupuncture, acupressure, heat or cold, massage or other non-drug modalities to help with pain
- Follow your care team's recommendations for restarting your usual medications and supplements. If you take medicines for blood pressure or blood sugar, monitor your pressure and sugars closely, as pain, other medications, and physiologic changes from stress or surgery can cause significant fluctuations and require short-term dose adjustments. Restarting

blood thinners for stroke prevention is particularly important so make sure your medical providers clearly advise you on when to resume these medicines

Copy this Post-Op Recovery Check list to guide you and your caregivers. Your surgical care team will also remind you of many of these points. However, the more you understand, the better prepared you are to work collaboratively with your care team.

Please review your notes, make sure you get all your questions answered, and have a nutritional strategy worked out in advance. Nutrition is foundational.

I included a couple bonus meditations to enjoy before and after surgery to support your recovery **Appendix 7**). I wish you the very best of health, a seamless surgery, and a swift recovery. I hope that you have implemented some permanent habit changes that will positively influence your health for the long-haul, helping you live an active and vibrant life.

CHAPTER 6
OPTIMIZING RECOVERY SUMMARY

- Continue plant-based diet and fiber to clear the colon
- Drink sufficient filtered water daily
- Organic coffee or dandelion/green/white tea to support kidney clearance of retained fluid
- Arnica orally and/or topically and Bromelian to help with bruising

- Walk around and sit up in a chair as much as you allowed
- Bathe or soak feet in warm water with Epsom salts to support detoxification through skin
- Continue deep breathing exercises at least hourly while awake (critical in the first 3 days after surgery to prevent pneumonia)
- Consider lymphatic massage or dry brushing for lymphatic support
- Continue support nutrients for at least 1 month post-op or until fully healed

Doctors won't make you healthy
Nutritionists won't make you slim
Teachers won't make you smart
Gurus won't make you calm
Mentors won't make you rich
Trainers won't make you fit
Ultimately, you have to take responsibility

Save yourself

Naval Ravikant

Chapter 7:

Vitality Beyond Surgery

By engaging in this program, you chose to be a proactive warrior rather than a passive victim. You committed to active stewardship of your health. I can assure you, the road less travelled offers a lifetime of difference.

In just a few chapters, I hope that you have developed an appreciation for the impact of lifestyle choices around diet, hydration, movement, stress management, attitude, and sleep on overall health. You understand the power of a positive mindset and strategies to replace unhealthy habits with those that will better serve your long-term health goals. I am hopeful you feel confident not only to face surgery but also to face virtually any health hazard, including cancer and aging, knowing that you possess powerful tools to navigate these unavoidable challenges.

I distilled for you many simple strategies that took me decades to learn and apply in my own life. I am optimistic, from witnessing the experiences of others, that your efforts will reward you not only with a successful surgery, but also with lifelong improved mood, energy, and vitality. Even the smallest habit change – giving up sodas, eating a vegetable-full salad/soup/chili/smoothie daily, cutting alcohol intake in half, and even just 5 minutes of exercise or meditative activity after brushing your teeth daily can have massive impact if you make these regular habits.

I also hope you eventually experience reduced reliance on medications by working with a proactive healthcare team that delves into the root causes of chronic ailments with a goal of preventing or reversing them. Our providers and health coaches have enjoyed helping many patients shed chronic disease. We believe our job is to help patients take problems off their problem lists and trim their medication lists. This preemptive, collaborative, goal-directed focus is the difference between "transformative care" and typical "pill-for-an-ill" medical care.

Life and health depend on our choices and daily habits. Devolving to instant gratification and short-term rescue mode leads to decades of chronic disease and disability, and is likely to rob you of years of vibrant life. Health need not be difficult or fraught with deprivation. Too many believe that being healthy is hard. In fact, nothing is more difficult than being chronically ill or disabled. To paraphrase Weight Watchers, nothing tastes as good as healthy feels. Remember, perfection is not the goal. I have a powerfully addictive sweet tooth and a tendency to self-soothe with chocolate. However, I have managed to set up my home, office and life to make healthy choices easy and I allow myself a daily healthy—but still delicious—low-carb or paleo treat, such as dark chocolate-covered almonds.

It is never too late to transform your health. I have witnessed brilliant health breakthroughs at every age. I hope that you continue to always treasure your health and return to this guide if you fall back into habits that fail you. I pray that you also experience amazement at the power of the human spirit and the miraculous healing power of the human body.

After all this complexity, I leave you with our simple vitality prescription— strategies for a long and healthy life:

LifeScape Vitality Prescription

- ❖ Breathe
- ❖ Eat mindfully and joyfully
- ❖ Laugh and play daily
- ❖ Immerse in nature
- ❖ Indulge in healthy sleep
- ❖ Enjoy nourishing movement
- ❖ Filter your inputs
- ❖ Treasure health, knowing that it is precious and fragile
- ❖ Invest in transformative care

Surgery relieves a symptom
Lifestyle prevents a replay

Appendix 1:

Am I A Good Surgical Candidate?

1. I am overweight or have accumulated
belly fat (waist > hips) — Y/N

2. I have trouble tolerating many medications — Y/N

3. I bruise or bleed easily or notice wounds
heal slowly — Y/N

4. I take more than 5 medicines daily or
any hormones, pain medicines, acid blockers,
or sleep medicines routinely — Y/N

5. I drink alcohol daily or ever drink heavily
(>4 for man, >3 for woman in a day) — Y/N

6. I smoke, vape or am regularly exposed
to passive tobacco — Y/N

7. I exercise less than 150 min (2 ½ hours)
per week — Y/N

8. I eat fewer than 3 servings of fruits
and vegetables daily — Y/N

9. I regularly consume sodas, processed foods,
sweets, or fast food — Y/N

10. I sleep poorly (<7hr per night), snore,
    or wake feeling groggy   Y/N

11. I have no daily routine or healthy strategy
    for managing stress   Y/N

12. I tend to think negatively, worry, or suffer
    anxious or depressed moods   Y/N

13. I have been told I have high blood
    pressure (>120/80), high blood sugar, insulin,
    A1c, or elevated liver enzymes   Y/N

14. I often feel fatigued or notice problems
    with memory, concentration/focus or brain fog   Y/N

15. I have difficulty breathing, asthma or
    chronic lung disease, or need to use inhalers
    at least weekly   Y/N

16. I have frequent digestive issues,
    heartburn, bloating, diarrhea or constipation,
    or bleeding   Y/N

Score 1 point for each YES

0-2   Excellent Health, keep up the good work

3-9   Average with room for improvement; select your top 3 areas to focus

>10   Significant Risk; defer surgery for at least 4 weeks, if possible, to work intensively on reducing your risks. Consider Functional medicine consult or consultation with a Functional Nutritionist/Health Coach (www.lifescapepremier.com)

Appendix 2:

Starting Point Metrics

Body Mass Index: _____

Waist/Hip Ratio: _____

Blood Pressure: _____
Fasting Blood Sugar/A1c: _____

hsCRP inflammatory marker: _____

Surgical Candidate Survey Score: _____

My Intention:_____

My Why – Committing to my health is crucial to me because:
_____
_____

And why is that?
_____
_____

And why is that?
_____
_____

"He who has a why can endure any how"

Friedrich Nietzche

Appendix 3:

Daily Habit Checklist

Morning Action Plan

- Review Your Intention and your Why
- Daily Mindfulness Meditation

Top Habit Action Items Today (be as specific as possible, i.e "I will walk for 30 minutes" or "I will eat a large salad today")

1. _____
2. _____
3. _____

Evening Gratitude Recap

- Check off and celebrate wins (habit action items successfully accomplished)
- For those that challenged, what tripped me up?
- What did I learn from trying that I could do differently next time?
- Daily journal, note:
    o Something that inspired me
    o Something that challenged me

- Something for which I am grateful
- Something that made me laugh
- Something that touched my heart

Remember small habit changes, practiced daily, even imperfectly, achieve massive results

Appendix 4:

Hidden Dangers In Your Medicine Cabinet

PPI Acid Blockers Omeprazole/Prilosec, Lasoprazole/Prevacid, Esomeprazole/Nexium, Dexlansoprazole/Dexilant, Rabeprazole/Aciphex and Pantoprazole/Protonix (some of which are OTC)

Recommended only for SHORT TERM treatment of acid reflux and occasionally longer term for more severe conditions. Chronic use of PPIs impairs absorption of many nutrients including calcium, magnesium and B vitamins, increases risk of fractures, pneumonia, C.difficile colitis, kidney disease, heart disease and dementia. PPIs may negate the heart benefits of Clopidogrel or Plavix blood thinner. Manage acid reflux by eating smaller meals (the majority of acid reflux results from eating too much—more food/drink than the stomach can handle). Also avoiding caffeine, alcohol, carbonation and chewing gum, fasting 3 hours before bed, elevating the head of your bed, juicing ¼ of a lemon in water once or twice daily, using melatonin or digestive bitters to promote motility, and going for a walk after meals helps prevent reflux and enhance digestion. Preferentially use shorter acting antacids like Maalox or Tums or H2 blockers like Famotidine only as needed (safely dispose of any Zantac or Ranitidine which was found to be a carcinogen). Getting off PPI medicines can be difficult as you may experience a rebound in acid. If interested, schedule an appointment with LifeScape Functional Nutritionists to walk you through a safe tapering process.

NSAIDs OTC Aspirin, Ibuprofen/Motrin/Advil, Naproxen/Aleve and prescription versions Etodolac/Lodine, Mobic, Celecoxib/Celebrex, Diclofenac/ Voltaren

Nsaids are responsible for more than 100,000 hospitalizations and 16,000 deaths annually in the US usually due to GI bleeding, cardiovascular events (high blood pressure, heart attack, stroke), and kidney failure. Nsaids increase bleeding risk and may impede bone healing. Avoid NSAIDs if taking diuretics, or have heart failure, kidney or liver disease, or when taking blood thinners or steroids like prednisone. Other Nsaids can impede the heart protective benefits of baby aspirin. Alcohol taken with Nsaids can further escalate risk of GI bleeding. Unless directed by your provider, most suggest stopping any NSAIDs a week prior to surgery.

TYLENOL acetaminophen; added to many over-the-counter cough and cold, migraine, and sleep medicines

Acetaminophen overdose is the leading cause for calls to Poison Control Centers (>100,000/year) and accounts for more than 56,000 emergency room visits, 2,600 hospitalizations, and at least 450 deaths due to acute liver failure each year. Acetaminophen is a potent liver toxin, especially dangerous when combined with alcohol. NEVER use acetaminophen for a hangover, effectively throwing an added toxin into an already poisoned liver. Never take more than 3000mg in 24hr, less if you are older or have impaired liver function. Those who drink alcohol daily, ever drink heavily, or take narcotics, hormones or statin medications should minimize Acetaminophen.

SLEEPING PILLS/SEDATING ANTIHISTAMINES

Sleeping pill use of any kind is associated with an increased risk of dying over 3-fold higher than in those who never take them. Cancer mortality is also higher, on par with smoking, in those taking sleeping pills, even sporadic use of as few as 18 tablets per year. Combining sleeping pills, including OTC Tylenol PM or benzodiazepine anxiety medicines with alcohol or narcotic pain relievers is particularly hazardous. Anyone with disrupted, un-refreshing sleep or witnessed snoring or breathing pauses should be evaluated for sleep apnea, breathing disruption while asleep, leading to dangerous oxygen deficit and a host of medical complications including atrial fibrillation, high blood pressure, heart attack/stroke, and early memory loss. Insomnia is best treated with sleep hygiene, unplugging from screens, and cognitive behavioral therapy. Sedating antihistamines, such as diphenhydramine, are associated with dry mouth, high blood pressure, eye pressure changes, urinary retention, constipation, falls, accidents, sleep apnea, confusion, and significantly higher risk of cognitive decline with long-term use.

HERBAL SUPPLEMENTS

Herbal products are chemically complex and very difficult to standardize, have the potential to interact with many medications, and some pose significant risk around surgery so they are best avoided for at least 2 weeks prior to surgery until fully healed. Products from China and India have potentially high rates of contamination with heavy metals or other toxic chemicals. Many, including Gingko Biloba, Garlic, Ginseng, Dong Quai, and Feverfew may increase bleeding risk. Ephedra and Garlic may increase blood pressure and cardiovascular risk. Kava is a potent liver toxin and should be avoided altogether. Kava, St. John's Wort, and Valerian root can interact with anesthetics during surgery and many herbal products including Echinacea and Goldenseal can interact with other medications commonly used around surgery.

Appendix 5:

Common Surgical Complications, Preventive Strategies, & When To Seek Help

INFECTIONS

Pneumonia (lung infections)

- ❖ Infections deep in the lungs are common after surgery due to shallow breathing (breathing that does not fully expand the lungs), lying in bed, and sedating medications that suppress your normal reflexes to cough or clear secretions. Pneumonia usually presents with fever, cough productive of discolored sputum, chills, drenching sweats, shortness of breath, wheezing, or pain with deep breaths
- ▪ ***Pneumonia Prevention Strategies***
    - Get vaccinated (see below)
    - Avoid any tobacco exposure before/after surgery
    - Avoid aerosols, fragrances or other lung irritants
    - Deep breathing frequently every hour to keep lungs open (if surgery involves the chest, splint with a pillow to minimize ribcage movement while fully expanding the lungs)

- o Use "The Breather" breathing trainer (available on Amazon) 10 deep in/out breaths dialed up to a challenging level to boost lung function BEFORE surgery
- Sit up & walk frequently once cleared to do so
- If asthmatic, make sure you have your rescue inhaler with you at all times to use as needed (request that you keep it at your bedside while in the hospital)
- Cough or use suction as needed to clear secretions
- Keep meals small & sit upright for at least an hour after meals
- Stay well hydrated and avoid dairy or sugary drinks
- Note: chronic use of acid blockers is associated with increased risk of pneumonia so reduce dependence on them prior to surgery if possible. Avoiding refined/processed foods, eating smaller meals, avoiding alcohol, carbonation, and caffeine, fasting 3hr before bed, and drinking lemon juice in water twice daily help reduce acid reflux symptoms

Bladder infections

❖ Infections of the bladder are common after surgery given frequent use of catheters and other factors. They usually present with pain during or after urination, sometimes fever or flank pain. They can sneak up on older patients without warning causing sudden confusion, fever, vomiting or diarrhea

- ***Bladder Infection Prevention Strategies***
  - Stay well-hydrated and urinate frequently
  - Avoid dietary bladder irritants, acidic foods, sugars, caffeine & alcohol
  - Consider D-Mannose supplement if prone to UTIs. D-mannose prevents one common bacteria from adhering to the lining of the bladder

Wound infections

❖ Infections of the surgical wound are always possible, no matter how sterile the procedure. Be alert and notify your medical team for increasing pain, redness, swelling, warmth, or any pus-like or foul-smelling discharge

- ***Preventing Wound Infections***
  - Follow surgeon's wound care instructions carefully
  - Stay well-hydrated
  - Eat healthy plant-based and fiber-rich diet avoiding refined or processed foods or added sugars
  - Eat foods rich in vitamin C and healthy proteins such as dark leafy greens, berries, citrus, bell peppers, and organic bone broths or whey protein
  - Wash hands frequently, keep fingernails trimmed, and use hand-sanitizer liberally especially while in hospital
  - Wipe down all frequently touched surfaces with antibacterial wipes or dilute bleach solution
  - Keep skin clean, dry, and well-moisturized to prevent cracking

Other infections

- Sepsis – system-wide infection in the blood stream, usually presenting with high fever and very acute illness requiring emergent care
- Dental – get a good dental check-up and cleaning at least a month prior to surgery; brush at least twice daily with soft toothbrush, floss or use a water pick daily, avoid antibacterial or alcohol-containing mouthwash
- Sinus – if prone to sinus infections, use saline rinses twice daily and eat anti-inflammatory diet avoiding dairy, sugars and refined starches/grains
- GI – gallbladder, pancreatitis, diverticulitis or appendicitis – notify your medical team of any fever with localized pain in the belly or back, nausea/vomiting, bleeding, jaundice, or change in bowel habits. Avoid alcohol before/after surgery until fully healed and off pain medications

A Word about VACCINATION:

- ❖ VACCINATION can significantly reduce your risk of pneumonia and whole body infections like sepsis and meningitis. Vaccination also serves to protect healthcare workers and other vulnerable patients in the hospital including the elderly, pregnant women, young children, or those whose immune systems are impaired
  - Particularly be sure to discuss with your physician:

- o Influenza vaccines during flu season especially if you are at high risk including any with lung or heart disease, diabetes, pregnancy, elderly or children
- o Pneumonia vaccines if over 65 or asthmatic, diabetic, or chronic heart, lung or kidney disease
- o Tetanus, ideally Tdap booster, within 5 years before any surgery
- o Hepatitis A and B vaccination is also a good idea prior to any hospital or surgical exposure
- o Given recent outbreaks of highly infectious diseases, make sure you are immune to measles and pertussis (Pertussis is in the Tdap booster)
- o Vaccines against bacterial meningitis are indicated before certain procedures including removal of the spleen
- o Ask about what vaccines should be considered for your special circumstances

SEEK IMMEDIATE HELP FOR:
- Fever
- Worsening pain/redness/swelling
- Shaking chills or drenching sweats
- Productive cough, pain with deep breath
- Shortness of breath
- Pain with urination

- Vomiting or diarrhea especially if with fever or pain
- Flank or abdominal pain with fever

DIGESTIVE COMPLICATIONS

❖ **Nausea/Vomiting** are common after surgery due to anesthesia and/or pain medicines slowing gut motility or just side effects of meds or the surgery itself

- *Preventing Nausea/Vomiting*
  - Inform your care team about any medication intolerances or preferences
  - Prior to surgery, if you have multiple sensitivities to medicines or any serious reactions, ask about genetic testing to learn more about how your body processes drugs. Pharmacogenetic Testing is available direct-to-consumer through companies like Genesight or 23 and me but medical interpretation with your primary care physician is encouraged to better understand them and use the results appropriately
  - Take ice chips or small sips of fluids initially
  - Ginger tea, chewing on candied ginger, or flat ginger ale can help settle an upset stomach
  - Keep the colon moving with adequate fluids, fiber, stool softeners, and laxatives as needed
  - If prone to nausea, bloating, or slow gut motility, nightly melatonin or aromatic bitters (brands include Bioceuticals Liposomal Bitters, Sweetish Bitters, or Iberogast) in a little water prior to eating supports moving food out of the stomach

- Sit up in a chair and walk as often as possible to promote motility

❖ **Diarrhea** is a common complication of antibiotic medicines often given during or after surgery. Anxiety, stimulants like caffeine, overactive thyroid, and other medication or supplement side effects can cause diarrhea
- *Preventing Diarrhea*
  - Support a healthy microbiome with a plant-based, fiber-rich diet avoiding refined/processed foods before surgery. Small amounts of daily fermented foods such as organic yogurt, kefir, kombucha, or fermented veggies help support a healthy gut microbiome (your immune defense and detoxification army)
  - Stay well-hydrated w/ filtered water, smoothies, & organic broths
  - Consider probiotics Saccharomyces boulardii and Lactobacillus rhamnosus / L. reuteri if antibiotics are used (always confirm with your medical team; avoid in extremely sick or immune-compromised patients)
  - Eat cooked and cooled rice, rice milk, applesauce, banana, bone broths and purees until diarrhea resolves. Avoid dairy, grains, legumes or roughage
  - Make sure the care team reevaluates medicines or supplements that might be causing diarrhea. Hold any non-essential supplements, including probiotics or magnesium, which might be triggering an adverse effect

- Only use anti-diarrheal medicines with medical guidance. Never use these medications if infectious diarrhea with fever or bleeding

❖ **Constipation** due to anesthetics, pain medicines and lack of mobility is extremely common and can be severe
- *Preventing Constipation*
  - Assure healthy gut motility before surgery by eating pant-based, fiber-rich diet. If necessary, use stool softeners (Colace or Docusate – agents that soften the stool) and laxatives (polyethylene glycol/Miralax, Dulcolax, senna, magnesium citrate or oxide – stimulants to move stool through faster) to clear the colon to achieve a good bowel movement daily
  - Magnesium citrate 200-400mg daily (caution if kidney disease). Hold if causing cramping or diarrhea
  - Consider fiber supplement and probiotics or small amounts of fermented foods like kefir, kombucha, yogurt, or fermented vegetables if tolerated
  - Stay well-hydrated
  - Sit up in chair and walk frequently as soon as cleared
  - Follow your medical team's guidance on constipation management

SEEK IMMEDIATE HELP FOR:
- Intractable vomiting, inability to keep fluids down
- Severe diarrhea or diarrhea with fever or bleeding
- Distention and inability to pass gas/stool

- Inability to have a bowel movement for over 2 days or pain/bleeding with passing a bowel movement

VASCULAR COMPLICATIONS

❖ **Bleeding** is a common risk after any surgery and some bleeding or bruising is to be expected. Your surgeon can tell you how much blood loss is normal and signs to be alert for to indicate excessive bleeding like feeling lightheaded on standing, becoming unusually pale or clammy, feeling faint or experiencing rapid heart rate or low blood pressure

- *Preventing bleeding complications*
  - In surgeries where bleeding risk is high, ask about autologous blood donation – giving your own blood in advance to transfuse if needed during or after surgery
  - Hold any medications or supplements that could increase bleeding risk prior to surgery:
    o *Ask your medical team to review necessity for aspirin or blood thinners* as stopping these or holding them too long, in certain instances, may be more risky than continuing them
    o Ask your medical team about alternatives for other medicines that increase bleeding risk including certain antidepressants (SSRIs/SNRAs) and all NSAID pain relievers (ibuprofen, naproxen, etc)

- *Stop fish oil, vitamin E, and herbal supplements including any with chondroitin, gingko, garlic, ginseng, dong quai, guarana, or feverfew at least a week prior to surgery*
- Follow your surgeon's post-operative instructions and activity restrictions to allow proper wound healing
- Keep wounds protected with sterile dressings
- Consider use of homeopathic arnica supplements topically or orally to support bruising resolution

❖ **Blood Clots** can occur at many sites including legs, abdomen or pelvis, lungs (called pulmonary emboli) or heart. Multiple factors cause risk for clots including surgical injury to blood vessels (triggering normal clotting processes), bedrest or lack of movement allowing blood to pool and clot, dehydration, infections such as Covid19, genetics, smoking, hormone medicines or other medical issues such as cancer

- *Preventing blood clots*
  - Know your risks in advance – particularly if you have any family history of blood clots or pulmonary emboli. Ask about advanced testing if any family history
  - Lose weight if possible prior to surgery
  - Make sure your provider reviews your medications and holds any that might cause clotting risk prior to surgery especially hormones
  - Avoid any tobacco exposure
  - Stay well-hydrated

- Move every body part often, walk when cleared
- Pump legs, calves frequently while lying in bed
- Wear support stockings to keep blood from pooling
- Deep breathing exercises frequently to keep lungs fully expanded and blood moving

❖ **Heart Attacks** can occur in those already at risk, given the stresses of surgery, fluid shifts or dehydration, or disruptions in breathing or blood flow. A heart attack usually presents with crushing chest pain or pain radiating to the jaw or left shoulder or through the back. Sometimes shortness of breath, sweaty or clammy feeling skin, or lightheadedness occur. ***Chest pain not relieved by antacids or position warrants immediate notification of your medical team***

❖ **Heart Rhythm Disorders** often complicate surgery and can lead to strokes or sudden death. Obesity, smoking, untreated sleep apnea, and heavy alcohol use increase the risk for these dangerous complications

- *Prevention of Heart Attacks and Heart Rhythm Disorders*
  - Eat a clean, heart healthy, plant-based Mediterranean diet prior to and after surgery, avoiding refined/processed foods, sugars, saturated fats and minimizing meats (make animal products a condiment)
  - If you snore or suffer from disrupted or non-refreshing sleep, request a sleep study to rule out sleep apnea. Untreated sleep apnea not only contributes to high blood sugar, accumulated belly fat, fatigue and difficulty

117

focusing, it dramatically worsens your risk of high blood pressure, heart attack, stroke, heart rhythm disorders like atrial fibrillation, and early dementia
- Avoid ANY tobacco or nicotine exposure for several weeks prior to surgery and until fully healed (ideally forever)
- Maintain an ideal weight; if obese or waist>hips, try to lose 10% of your weight before surgery
- Avoid prolonged sitting and engage in physical activity daily before and as soon as possible after surgery
- Stay well-hydrated so your urine appears pretty clear
- Deep breathing every hour while awake
- If taking blood thinners for atrial fibrillation, make sure your physician confirms the minimum amount of time, if any, you can be off them safely around surgery and when to resume them

❖ **Fluid Retention/Swelling** is common after surgery due to IV fluids given during the procedure or fluid shifts triggered by bedrest, poor lymphatic or venous flow, and wound healing. Conditions like heart failure, varicose veins, or chronic venous insufficiency aggravated by obesity, thyroid disease, or certain medications also contribute

- *Prevention of fluid retention/swelling*
  - Achieve as close to a healthy weight prior to surgery
  - Request comprehensive thyroid and kidney testing if prone to swelling/fluid retention

- Follow healthy plant-based diet avoiding refined/processed foods and added sugars or salt
- Consume more diuretic foods such as dandelion, nettle, mint, or hibiscus tea, green or white tea, watermelon, asparagus, lemons, cucumber, celery
- Use support stockings or sequential venous compression devices to keep blood moving after surgery
- Elevate legs above heart level when at rest
- Consider investing in lymphatic massage if prone to fluid retention

SEEK IMMEDIATE HELP FOR:
- Acute shortness of breath
- Pain with deep breath
- Crushing chest pain
- Pain radiating to jaw or left arm or back
- Feeling faint or lightheaded
- Looking pale, sweaty or clammy
- Palpitations or heart racing, especially if lightheaded, short of breath, or chest heaviness
- Swelling or calf pain in one limb

RESPIRATORY COMPLICATIONS

❖ **Shortness of breath** is common especially after recovering from a lengthy procedure or one involving the chest or abdomen. Anxiety can also trigger shortness of breath

- ❖ **Asthma/Chronic Lung Disease** can flare from exposure to anesthesia, chemicals and inhalants in the operating room or hospital and the stress of undergoing surgery
  - *Prevention of Respiratory Complications*
    - See pneumonia prevention strategies above
    - If prone to lung disease or any tobacco exposure, even remotely, make sure to have baseline lung function testing prior to surgery and inform your surgeon and anesthesiologist of your status, triggers/sensitivities, and medications used
    - Avoid exposure to any tobacco, dust, pollutants, fragrances, or heavy pollens prior to surgery
    - Defer surgery if experiencing a symptom flare or possible infection
    - Bring your medications to the hospital and request that you keep your rescue inhaler at your bedside for use as needed
    - Practice relaxing breathing meditation and 3-4 deep breaths several times a day leading up to surgery and while in the hospital
    - If concerned about your lung function, use a training device such as The Breather (available online), sing, or play a wind instrument to help strengthen your lung function
    - Use a pillow or your hand to splint painful areas while allowing full deep breaths after surgery
    - Sit up in a chair and walk as much as possible to allow lungs to fully expand

- Let nursing staff know if surgical dressings are too tight or constricting breathing

NEUROLOGIC COMPLICATIONS

- ❖ **Headaches or Confusion/Dizziness/Brain Fog** often occur due to stress, fatigue, pain, dehydration, or as a consequence of anesthesia or other medications
  - ▪ *Prevention of Headaches, Confusion, Dizziness, Brain Fog*
    - Eat a healthy plant-based, organic diet rich in fiber and fruits/veggies for several weeks leading up to surgery
    - Drink at least one or two green drinks or smoothies daily after surgery
    - Take fiber and supplements to support liver clearance of toxins
    - Avoid alcohol, Tylenol or other liver toxins
    - If prone to adverse drug reactions, ask about genetic testing to learn more about how your body processes drugs. Pharmacogenetic Testing is available direct-to-consumer through companies like Genesight or 23andme but medical interpretation with your primary care physician is encouraged to better understand them and use the results appropriately
    - Stay well-hydrated so that your urine looks pretty clear

- ❖ **Strokes or TIAs** can occur in those with vascular disease risks. Preventive strategies are the same as those above for heart attacks or heart rhythm disorders

SEEK IMMEDIATE HELP FOR:

- Headache, confusion, severe lightheadedness, or any focal complaints like weakness, numbness, or problems with speech, balance, facial weakness, or vision

SKIN COMPLICATIONS

- ❖ The skin is a critical protective organ that is frequently traumatized in the surgical process by application of harsh chemicals, surgical incisions, repeated pokes for IVs and blood draws. As a crucial barrier to infection, it is imperative we treat the skin to extra TLC around surgery
- ❖ **Rashes** are common from exposure to skin cleansers, bandages, wound dressings, shaving areas, hospital linens, latex gloves, catheters, and reactions to medications, foods, or supplements
- ❖ **Bed sores/skin ulcerations** occur mainly in those with very poor nutritional status, smokers, or severely weak, bed-ridden, or elderly
- *Prevention of skin disorders after surgery*
    - Eat a nutritious plant-based diet rich in healthy fats, proteins, and foods rich in vitamin C
    - Avoid refined starches, sugars and processed foods
    - Use hypoallergenic organic skin care products (soaps, lotions, and laundry products) as much as possible
    - Notify staff of any allergies to latex, adhesives or bandages, iodine or other topical agents

- Keep skin clean, dry, and moisturized with hypo-allergenic, fragrance free creams with ceramides such as Cerave, Aveeno, or Cetaphil
- Request special bed or mattress pad to prevent pressure sores and make sure to move and change position frequently
- Get up and move as often as possible to help blood flow
- Make sure any cracked skin or rashes, pressure points or sores are treated promptly

Appendix 6:

Mindset For Intention

Setting our intention is the most critical step in achieving our health goals. Too often, we careen through life mindlessly and take our health for granted.

When patients ask me "WHY did this happen?" I often reflect on how miraculous is it that the body works as well as it does given how we treat ourselves day after day.

We fill our bodies with junk, fail to recharge or move, and live constantly stressed and overwhelmed.

We get mired in the toxic emotions of shame, blame, criticism, and complaint.

You reap what you focus on, so mindfully shift your focus towards a healing mindset. Happiness is a verb, attitude is a choice, and gratefulness is your action plan.

So let's take a few moments each day to slow down, take some deep breaths, and indulge in gratefulness for this amazing vessel of the human body, including those areas that maybe are not working so well.

Get comfortable, close your eyes, let your hands rest gently in your lap, and allow your muscles to relax in your face, your neck and shoulders, your back and torso, arms/hands, and legs/feet – giving thanks for the incredible work each part does every day.

Breathe in and out, committing to clearing away negative thoughts and inputs that don't serve you.

Breathe in and out, committing to treasuring health and providing what you know your body needs to heal.

Breathe in and experience gratitude for the wonders of modern medicine and brilliant healers that provide hope for healing.

Breathe in gratitude for your supporters – friends, family, co-workers, clergy, therapists, etc – everyone supporting your journey to health.

Breathe in and appreciate the brilliant power of your own mind, body, and spirit to heal and thrive.

Say, "I am committed to honoring myself by treasuring my health and not taking a single day for granted."

Appendix 7:

Meditation Before Surgery

Sit comfortably, close your eyes, and take several deep, cleansing breaths, feeling the breath enter the nostrils and fill your chest all the way down into your belly.

Allow yourself to imagine entering the operating room in a state of gratitude as you recite the following mantra:

I am calm and confident that all will go well and that I will heal quickly and fully.

I am calm and confident that all will go well and that I will heal quickly and fully.

I am calm and confident that all will go well and that I will heal quickly and fully.

I breathe in a deep breath of gratitude for the devoted care of my surgical team who will support me through this journey.

I breathe in gratitude for the technology and expertise developed over centuries that allows me to heal.

I breathe in gratefulness for all who will support me through my recovery.

I breathe in profound gratitude for the incredible healing power of my body – for the tissues that miraculously mend when damaged, the immune cells that fend off infection, destroy cancer cells, and promote healing, and even for the nervous system that signals pain or distress so that I may pay attention to these and take the proper steps to support my body.

I breathe in pride for the care I have taken to ensure I am in the best possible condition to undergo an operation.

I am calm and confident that all will go well and that I will heal quickly and fully.

I am calm and confident that all will go well and that I will heal quickly and fully.

Meditation After Surgery

Sit or lie comfortably, taking several deep, cleansing breaths through your nose.

Notice the breath as it enters the nostrils, fills the chest, and flows all the way down into the belly.

Feel the breath move life-supporting oxygen to your entire body, out to the very tips of your fingers and toes, especially to any injured parts, and then, just as quickly, feel the breath as it clears out spent air and any residual toxins your body no longer needs.

Notice how each breath, like waves on the beach, flows naturally and comfortably, entering and leaving quietly.

Notice any pain or discomfort, understanding that pain is an important signal that your body is injured, calling on your immune system's miraculous healers to come to the rescue and engage in healing the injury.

Take deep cleansing breaths, splinting painful areas if need be, and allow the breath to gently enter the injured area, bringing critical oxygen and blood flow to healing tissues.

Imagine your breath energizing your immune cells so that they can vigilantly contain and remove infections or wayward cancer cells while engaging in repair.

Notice any feelings of fear or anxiety, understanding these are normal.

Breathe into the anxiousness, allowing a moment of peace, and allow anxious thoughts to drift by like clouds in the sky.

Breathe in gratitude for your care team and all those supporting your recovery. Breathe in gratitude for the facilities and technology that support miraculous healing.

Breathe in gratitude for your own brilliant healing power, and the hard work you performed to support your healthy recovery.

Breathe in gratitude for your WHY—the reasons that treasuring your health became a priority to you.

Breathe in gratitude for living to see another day, vowing never to take another day for granted.

Appendix 8:

Resources For Additional Support

Could you benefit from a Functional Medicine Consultation?

Once upon a time, I thought I was healthy, but I was actually a hot mess. Chronically tired, in chronic pain. I felt 100 years old as I got out of bed every morning because every joint was stiff and sore. Functional medicine saved my life and revived my health. If you also feel like a hot mess, then you might benefit from a functional medicine consult.

Our functional medicine consult involves a comprehensive history, a timeline of your symptoms over the course of your entire lifetime, even back before you were born, and influences that might have affected your health from when your mom was pregnant with you. We look into your genetics and your family history. We consider advanced testing that might help us really get to the underlying causes of your chronic symptoms. As cost effectively as possible, we might evaluate for nutrient deficiency, food or food additive sensitivity, environmental toxins, gut microbial imbalances, genetic testing or functional testing showing how well your body operates. Then we pull this all together and collaborate with you on an action plan to address those root causes and tackle them once and for all.

For one recent patient, we literally took 11 medical problems off of a list that had been plaguing her for 40-plus years and eliminated all five of her chronic high-risk medications. It is possible to actually uncover and resolve chronic diseases I previously thought unresolvable, including attention deficit disorder, chronic fatigue, arthritis (including rheumatoid arthritis), autoimmune disorders, type 2 diabetes, and even cognitive impairment. So, if you scored over 10 on the *Am I a Good Surgical Candidate* quiz or you are simply sick and tired of feeling sick and tired, book a Functional Medicine consultation with us at www.lifescapepremier.com and watch your life change immeasurably.

Do You Need Added Support from a Nutritionist/Health Coach?

If you need extra guidance or support to shift your diet in a healthy direction, then consider booking a consultation with functional medicine-certified nutritionists / health coaches. Online or in-person appointments are available to help you evaluate your diet and health habits and uncover some simple tweaks that, over time, could improve your health dramatically. Our nutritionists go into great depth and offer very personalized support. Nutrition is, without a doubt, one of the most critical and fundamental ways to achieve your health goals, but it is a tremendous struggle for all of us in this *obesogenic* world. Do not hesitate to book a consultation with one of our nutritionists at www.lifescapepremier.com to create a personalized program for achieving your health goals.

Do You Need Extra Fitness or Myofascial Help?

If you have no idea where to begin to get back to fitness after years of being sedentary, in chronic pain, or limited by injury, then I encourage you to schedule a consultation with our fitness coach or work closely with a physical therapist. LifeScape's fitness coach can work personally with you, virtually or in-person, developing a program, working around your injuries or your disabilities, with a goal towards restoring your health.

Our bodies need to move. Every joint, every muscle needs to move. When we fail to move properly, our muscles become lax and our joints become unstable or stiff and painful. If you are not moving, you are decaying, so I encourage you to engage with our fitness coach and get a little extra help getting you on your way to achieving your fitness goals.

For extra myofascial support, consider a virtual consult with my "body whisperer" at sterlingstructuraltherapy.com.

131

Other Resources (U.S.)

Environmental Working Group ewg.org

Dirty Dozen/Clean Fifteen food list

Healthy living APP for green/clean products for home, skin care

Tap water database of environmental toxins in your water supply

Surgeon Rating:

Note: Physician ratings should be taken with a grain of salt, as they do not account for the baseline health or socioeconomic status of the surgeon's patient population or their patient's baseline case complexity or complication risk

Surgeon Scorecard:

https://abouthealthtransparency.org/re-port-card-directory/national-report-cards/surgeon-scorecard-propublica/

Hospital Ratings:

Hospital Safety Grade

https://www.hospitalsafetygrade.org/your-hospitals-safety-grade

Medicare CMS Hospital Compare

www.medicare.gov/hospitalcompare

Healthcare Service Pricing Comparison:

Healthcare Bluebook APP

https://www.healthcarebluebook.com/

Drug Pricing & Discount Guides:

GoodRX Drug Pricing https://www.goodrx.com/

Needy Meds Drug Pricing

https://www.needymeds.org/drug-pricing

Appendix 9:

Simple Healing Recipes

Simple Healing Recipes

SYSTEM for SIMPLE SCRUMPTIOUS SUPER-HEALING FOODS

Basic Concepts

- ☑ Remember the 5 "S's" to boost veggie intake toward your goal of 5-9 cups daily:
  Smoothies, **S**oups, **S**alads, **S**tews/Chilis, **S**tir-fries/Bowls
- ☑ Aim for fresh or frozen, organic, non-GMO ingredients
- ☑ Change it up – a diverse diet provides more nutrients, less chance of triggering allergic reactions
- ☑ Keep it clean - avoid added sugars, artificial sweeteners, preservatives, processed foods
- ☑ If you MUST sweeten, use a little raw honey, maple syrup, or Stevia
- ☑ Get creative and HAVE FUN combining ingredients or adding herbs, spices, flavorings
- ☑ Keep it SIMPLE by prepping all your veggies on one day a week – make it a family affair
- ☑ Make large batches and freeze ahead in glass containers for easy meals later

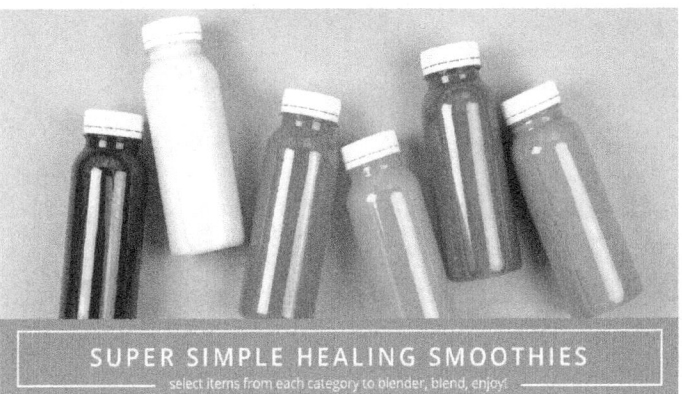

SUPER SIMPLE HEALING SMOOTHIES
select items from each category to blender, blend, enjoy!

1-1/12 Cups of LIQUID	1+c VEGGIES	2T HEALTHY FAT	1-2 FRUIT Servings	PROTEIN
Filtered water	Greens: spinach, kale, Swiss chard	MCT/coconut oil	Berries- all types – 1 cup	2 Tablespoons Nut butter
Greens drink	Cucumber	Avocado/oil	Apple - 1	1 tablespoon Peanut Butter Powder
Tea or Kombucha	Beet	Nut butter	½ cup Mango	
Coconut water	Carrot	Ground flaxseed	Banana	2 Tablespoons Flax/ Chia /Hemp Seeds
Non-dairy milks	Zucchini/ Celery	Chia seed	Acai/Pomegranate	1/2c Silken Tofu
Grassfed Milk	Cauliflower	Grassfed ghee	Citrus – 1 Orange	1/2c Yogurt/Kefir
Sheep/Goat Milk	Canned Unsweetened Pumpkin/Squash		Melon	½ cup Cottage cheese
			Dates – 1-2 pieces	Protein powder*

135

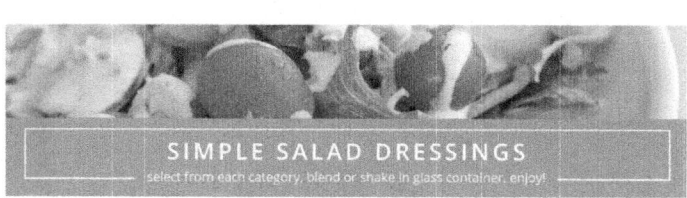

SIMPLE SALAD DRESSINGS
select from each category, blend or shake in glass container, enjoy!

3 parts OIL (3 Tablespoons)	1 part ACID (1 Tablespoon)	FLAVORINGS
Extra Virgin Olive	Vinegar Apple Cider Vinegar	1 clove Roasted crushed garlic
Avocado	Citrus Juice – Lemons, Limes or Oranges	1 tsp Ginger
Grapeseed	Wine	2+T Minced herbs/parsley/basil/tarragon/dill
Almond/Walnut/Hazelnut		1t Citrus Zest
Organic Canola		1T Dijon mustard
		Crushed Peppers/Sriracha
		1t honey or pinch of sugar

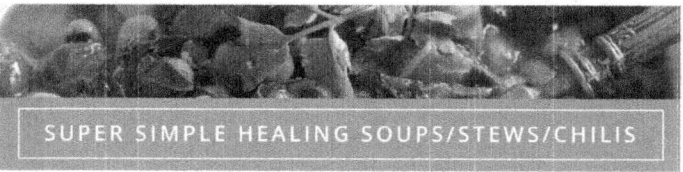

SUPER SIMPLE HEALING SOUPS/STEWS/CHILIS

Add items to large soup or Crock pot, heat & simmer, adjusting fluid amount to make soup vs stew / chili, salt lightly to taste

4-8c LIQUID BASE	4-6c VEGGIES	1-2c PROTEIN	HERBS/SPICES	1c GRAIN
Vegetable broth	Diced/sautéed onion	Lentils	Garlic	Wild Rice
Chicken broth	Diced/sautéed carrot	Beans	Parsley	Barley
Beef Bone Broth	Diced celery	Diced Poultry	Minced herbs	Brown Rice
Miso Broth	Cubed potato, yam	Diced Beef	Cilantro	Quinoa
Ham hock	Diced Parsnip/Jicama	Diced Ham	Ginger	Faux Rice: Cauliflower
Coconut Milk	Peas/Snow peas	Sausage	Peppers/chili sauce	Zoodles
	Diced tomato	Shrimp/Crab	Citrus Zest/juice	Rice Noodles
	Shredded Cabbage			Gluten Free Pasta/Noodles
	Greens (add at end)			

Simple Healing Recipes

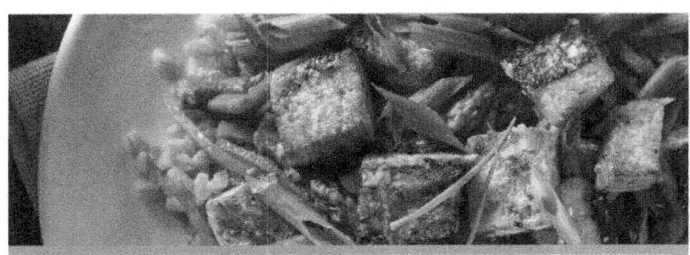

SUPER SIMPLE HEALING STIR-FRYS/BOWLS

Prep everything into bite size pieces. Either precook & throw together in a bowl or saute, w/minced garlic/ ginger in very hot wok or pot starting w/ protein, then veggies. Serve over cooked grain. Simplest stir fry sauce*: blend 1/4c liquid aminos/soy sauce, 1/4c broth, 1T sesame oil, 2T rice vinegar, 1 T cornstarch or arrowroot powder. Use to marinade your meat first or add sauce toward the end of stir fry. Add crushed red pepper if desired.

1-2c PROTIEN	3-4c VEGGIES	2T OIL	SAUCE	2c COOKED GRAIN
Diced Poultry	Diced onions	Canoia	Soy or aminos*	Brown/Black rice
Diced Meat	Sliced cabbage	Avocado	Curry	Quinoa
Beans/Lentils	Diced carrots	Grapeseed	Vinaigrette	Couscous
Edamame/Tofu	Diced zucchini	Peanut	Citrus	Noodles
Wild Shrimp	Diced squash		Garlic	
	Sliced Bok choy		Wine	
	Sliced radish		Salad dressings	
	Diced potato			
	Shredded greens			
	Diced asparagus			
	Diced celery			

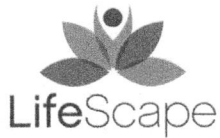

137

References

American Society of Anesthesiologists Task Force on Acute Pain Management. Practice guidelines for acute pain management in the perioperative setting: an updated report by the American Society of Anesthesiologists Task Force on Acute Pain Management. Anesthesiology. 20121162248-273.

Ahmad T, et al, Use of failure-to-rescue to identify international variation in postoperative care in low-, middle- and high-income countries: a 7-day cohort study of elective surgery. Br J Anaesth, 2017 Aug 1;119(2):258-266.

Barletta J F, Asgeirsson T, Senagore A J. Influence of intravenous opioid dose on postoperative ileus. Ann Pharmacother. 2011; 45(7-8):916–923.

Brennan F, Carr D B, Cousins M. Pain management: a fundamental human right. Anesth Analg. 2007;105(1):205–221.

Chung K, Kotsis S, Complications in Surgery: Root Cause Analysis and Preventive Measures. PLoS One. 2016; 11(3): e0150367.

Dajani E Z, Islam K. Cardiovascular and gastrointestinal toxicity of selective cyclo-oxygenase-2 inhibitors in man. J Physiol Pharmacol. 2008;59 02:117–133.

De Oliveira G S Jr, Agarwal D, Benzon H T. Perioperative single dose ketorolac to prevent postoperative pain: a meta-analysis of randomized trials. Anesth Analg. 2012;114(2):424–433.

Garimella V, Cellini C, Postoperative Pain Control. Clin Colon Rectal Surg. 2013 Sep; 26(3): 191–196.

Hodges R, Minich D, Modulation of Metabolic Detoxification Pathways Using Foods and Food-Derived Components: A Scientific Review with Clinical Application. J Nutr Metab. 2015; 2015: 760689.

Healey M, et al, Complications in Surgical Patients. Arch Surg, 2002, May: 137(5):611-7.

Huddleston, Peggy, *Prepare for Surgery, Heal Faster: A Guide to Mind-Body Techniques.* Angel River Press. 1996

Hugate R, Holland R, *The Handbook of Hip & Knee Joint Replacement, Through the Eyes of the Patient, Surgeon, & Medical Team.* Self-published. 2012.

Kehlet H, Jensen T S, Woolf C J. Persistent postsurgical pain: risk factors and prevention. Lancet. 2006; 367(9522): 1618–1625. [PubMed] [Google Scholar]

Komastu S, et al, Efficacy of perioperative synbiotics treatment for the prevention of surgical site infection after laparoscopic colorectal surgery: a randomized controlled trial. Surg Today. 2016; 46:479-490

Kotzampassi K et al, A four probiotics regimen reduces postoperative complications after colorectal surgery: a randomized, double-blind, placebo-controlled study. World J Surg. 2015; 39:2776-2783

Liu K et al, 'Probiotics' effects on the incidence of nosocomial pneumonia in critically ill patients: a systemic review and meta-analysis. Crit Care. 2012;16:R109

139

Maund E, McDaid C, et al, Paracetamol and selective and non-selective non-steroidal anti-inflammatory drugs for the reduction in morphine-related side-effects after major surgery: a systematic review. Br J Anaesth. 2011;106(3):292–297.

Nestor, James, *Breath: The New Science of a Lost Art*, Riverhead Books, 2020

Patil S, Sen S, Bral M, et al, Role of Acupuncture in Pain Management. Curr Pain Headache Rep. 2016 Apr;20(4):22.

Ralls M et al, Intestinal microbial diversity and perioperative complications. J Parenteral Enteral Nutrition. 2014; 38:392-399.

Schug S A, Raymann A. Postoperative pain management of the obese patient. Best Pract Res Clin Anaesthesiol. 2011;25(1):73–81.

Stavreau G, Kotzampassi K, Gut Microbiome, surgical complications, and probiotics. Ann Gastroenterol. 2017; 30(1): 45-53.

The International Surgical Outcomes Study group, Update/Correction: Global patient outcomes after elective surgery: prospective cohort study in 27 low-, middle- and high-income countries. Br J Anaesth. 2017 September; 119(3): 553.

The International Surgical Outcomes Study Group, Global patient outcomes after elective surgery: prospective cohort study in 27 low-, middle- and high-income countries, *British Journal of Anaesthesia*, Volume 117, Issue 5, November 2016, Pages 601–609

Toms L, McQuay H J, Derry S, Moore R A. Single dose oral paracetamol (acetaminophen) for postoperative pain in adults. Cochrane Database Syst Rev. 2008;(4):CD004602. [PMC free article][PubMed] [Google Scholar]

Wu M-S, Chen K-S, et.al., The Efficacy of Acupuncture in Post-Operative Pain Management: A Systematic Review and Meta-Analysis. Evid Based Complement Alternat Med. 2017

Xiang A, Cheng K, et al., The Immediate Analgesic Effect of Acupuncture for Pain: A Systematic Review and Meta-Analysis. Published online 2017 Oct 25.

Zafar N, Davies R, Greenslade G L, Dixon A R. The evolution of analgesia in an 'accelerated' recovery programme for resectional laparoscopic colorectal surgery with anastomosis. Colorectal Dis. 2010;12(2):119–124.

Acknowledgements

I owe profound gratitude to every patient who honored me with their most important asset, their health. Each patient's challenges, questions, encouragement, and knowledge helped me become a wiser physician and better human being.

I will forever be grateful for my education, which I am fortunate to pay forward every day, and for all the mentors in my career, from my teachers and colleagues at Punahou School in Honolulu, Washington University in St. Louis, the George Washington School of Medicine in Washington D.C., the United States Air Force Medical Corps, and the Mayo Clinic. I will be forever grateful to all the innovative providers who helped create our revolutionary patient-centered dream practice, LifeScape, especially Drs. William Strohman and Laurie Pozun who embraced my vision from the outset, brought our dream to life, and continue inspiring brilliant health breakthroughs every day.

A special thank-you to Drs. Jeffrey Bland and Mark Hyman for sparking the revolutionary movement, Functional Medicine (ifm.org), that shattered failing paradigms, salvaged my health and provided us with a novel operating system to move beyond "chronic disease management" to inspire and empower meaningful health transformation.

I hold boundless appreciation for my family, who never cease to inspire, support, and challenge me. To my brilliant daughters who motivate me to heal the world. Special thanks for my husband, Robert, my self-appointed "accommodator" who believed in me especially when I doubted myself, and whose relentless support gives our dreams wings.

About The Author

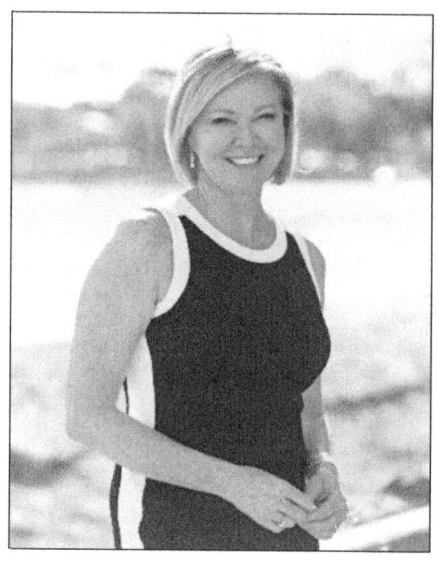

Susan Wilder, MD, IFMCP, is the co-founder and CEO of LifeScape, an award-winning Family Medicine practice dedicated to inspiring and empowering health transformation. Dr. Wilder received her Bachelor of Arts in Biology and Psychology from Washington University in St. Louis, Missouri and her medical degree from The George Washington University in Washington, DC. Dr. Wilder completed her specialty training in Family Medicine at Andrews Air Force Base, Maryland where she eventually became Assistant Chairman of the Department of Family Medicine. Following her military service, including deployment to Africa for Operation Restore Hope, Dr. Wilder relocated to Scottsdale, Arizona where she served as founding Director of the Mayo Clinic Scottsdale's Family Medicine Residency.

Dr. Wilder is Board-Certified in Family Medicine and a Certified Functional Medicine Practitioner. She earned a Certificate of Added Qualifications in Sports Medicine, has advanced training in Clinical Genomics, completed a fellowship in Faculty Development at the University of North Carolina at Chapel Hill, and attended the Air Force's School of Aerospace Medicine. She studied meditation with Deepak Chopra, brain health with Dr. Daniel Amen, human motivation with Tony Robbins, and Functional Medicine with Drs. Mark Hyman, Jeffrey Bland and the IFM faculty. Dr. Wilder has served as faculty for the Uniformed Services University of the Health Sciences, The George Washington University School of Medicine and Health Sciences, the Mayo Clinic College of Medicine, the University of Arizona College of Medicine, and the Southwest College of Naturopathic Medicine.

She is married to her husband, Robert, whom she met on her first day of college. Together they raised three brilliant daughters, and at least as many golden retrievers. She practices what she preaches, engaging in rituals including daily meditation, regular exercise such as yoga and hiking, and enjoys cooking a mostly healthy (sweet tooth not withstanding) plant-based diet.

Made in the USA
Monee, IL
10 March 2021